Keith M. Kilty
Elizabeth A. Segal
Editors

Rediscovering the Other America: The Continuing Crisis of Poverty and Inequality in the United States

Rediscovering the Other America: The Continuing Crisis of Poverty and Inequality in the United States has been co-published simultaneously as *Journal of Poverty*, Volume 7, Numbers 1/2 2003.

Pre-publication
REVIEWS,
COMMENTARIES,
EVALUATIONS...

"AN EXTREMELY IMPORTANT BOOK for social scientists, social workers, and healthcare practitioners."

Tony Tripodi, DSW
Dean and Professor,
College of Social Work,
The Ohio State University

Rediscovering the Other America: The Continuing Crisis of Poverty and Inequality in the United States

Rediscovering the Other America: The Continuing Crisis of Poverty and Inequality in the United States has been co-published simultaneously as *Journal of Poverty*, Volume 7, Numbers 1/2 2003.

The *Journal of Poverty* Monographic "Separates"

Below is a list of "separates," which in serials librarianship means a special issue simultaneously published as a special journal issue or double-issue *and* as a "separate" hardbound monograph. (This is a format which we also call a "DocuSerial.")

"Separates" are published because specialized libraries or professionals may wish to purchase a specific thematic issue by itself in a format which can be separately cataloged and shelved, as opposed to purchasing the journal on an on-going basis. Faculty members may also more easily consider a "separate" for classroom adoption.

"Separates" are carefully classified separately with the major book jobbers so that the journal tie-in can be noted on new book order slips to avoid duplicate purchasing.

You may wish to visit Haworth's website at . . .

http://www.HaworthPress.com

. . . to search our online catalog for complete tables of contents of these separates and related publications.

You may also call 1-800-HAWORTH (outside US/Canada: 607-722-5857), or Fax 1-800-895-0582 (outside US/Canada: 607-771-0012), or e-mail at:

docdelivery@haworthpress.com

Rediscovering the Other America: The Continuing Crisis of Poverty and Inequality in the United States, edited by Keith M. Kilty, PhD, and Elizabeth A. Segal, PhD (Vol. 7, No. 1/2, 2003). *"AN EXTREMELY IMPORTANT BOOK for social scientists, social workers, and healthcare practitioners."* (Tony Tripodi, DSW, Dean and Professor, College of Social Work, The Ohio State University)

Latino Poverty in the New Century: Inequalities, Challenges and Barriers, edited by Maria Vidal de Haymes, PhD, Keith M. Kilty, PhD, and Elizabeth A. Segal, PhD (Vol. 4, No. 1/2, 2000). *Provides social workers and policymakers with wide-ranging analyses of some of the pressing issues and social policies that highlight the impact of inequality and poverty in relation to available resources and opportunities.*

Pressing Issues of Inequality and American Indian Communities, edited by Elizabeth A. Segal, PhD, and Keith M. Kilty, PhD (Vol. 2, No. 4, 1998). *"Useful in its illustrations of the different impact of social welfare policy on diverse communities. . . . An important and valuable resource."* (Sandra S. Butler, PhD, Associate Professor, School of Social Work, University of Maine)

Income Security and Public Assistance for Women and Children, edited by Keith M. Kilty, PhD, Virginia E. Richardson, PhD, MSW, and Elizabeth A. Segal, PhD, MSW (Vol. 1, No. 2, 1997). *"Offers valuable insight and direction for ensuring income security and public assistance for women and children who are in poverty and gives them an opportunity to present what they believe they need to have in order to become independent."* (American Public Welfare Association)

Rediscovering the Other America: The Continuing Crisis of Poverty and Inequality in the United States

Keith M. Kilty
Elizabeth A. Segal
Editors

Rediscovering the Other America: The Continuing Crisis of Poverty and Inequality in the United States has been co-published simultaneously as *Journal of Poverty*, Volume 7, Numbers 1/2 2003.

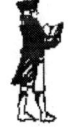

The Haworth Press, Inc.
New York • London • Oxford

Rediscovering the Other America: The Continuing Crisis of Poverty and Inequality in the United States has been co-published simultaneously as *Journal of Poverty*™, Volume 7, Numbers 1/2 2003.

© 2003 by The Haworth Press, Inc. All rights reserved. No part of this work may be reproduced or utilized in any form or by any means, electronic or mechanical, including photocopying, microfilm and recording, or by any information storage and retrieval system, without permission in writing from the publisher. Printed in the United States of America.

The development, preparation, and publication of this work has been undertaken with great care. However, the publisher, employees, editors, and agents of The Haworth Press and all imprints of The Haworth Press, Inc., including The Haworth Medical Press® and Pharmaceutical Products Press®, are not responsible for any errors contained herein or for consequences that may ensue from use of materials or information contained in this work. Opinions expressed by the author(s) are not necessarily those of The Haworth Press, Inc. With regard to case studies, identities and circumstances of individuals discussed herein have been changed to protect confidentiality. Any resemblance to actual persons, living or dead, is entirely coincidental.

Cover design by Jennifer Gaska

Library of Congress Cataloging-in-Publication Data

Rediscovering the other America : the continuing crisis of poverty and inequality in the United States / edited by Keith M. Kilty and Elizabeth A. Segal.
    p. cm.
    "Co-published simultaneously as Journal of poverty, volume 7, numbers 1/2, 2003."
    Includes bibliographical references and index.
    ISBN 0-7890-2096-3 (hard : alk. paper)–ISBN 0-7890-2097-1 (soft : alk. paper)
    1. Poor–Services for–United States. 2. Public welfare–United States. 3. Social policy–United States. I. Kilty, Keith M. (Keith Michael), 1946- II. Segal, Elizabeth A. III. Journal of poverty.
HV4045 .R38 2003
362.5'0973–dc21

2003001532

Indexing, Abstracting & Website/Internet Coverage

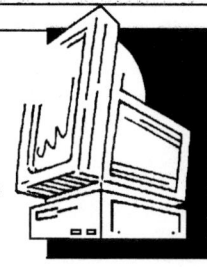

This section provides you with a list of major indexing & abstracting services. That is to say, each service began covering this periodical during the year noted in the right column. Most Websites which are listed below have indicated that they will either post, disseminate, compile, archive, cite or alert their own Website users with research-based content from this work. (This list is as current as the copyright date of this publication.)

Abstracting, Website/Indexing Coverage	Year When Coverage Began
• *Alzheimer's Disease Education & Referral Center (ADEAR)*	1997
• *Applied Social Sciences Index & Abstracts (ASSIA) (Online: ASSI via Data-Star) (CDRom: ASSIA Plus) <www.csa.com>*	1997
• *CNPIEC Reference Guide: Chinese National Directory of Foreign Periodicals*	1997
• *Criminal Justice Abstracts*	1997
• *Educational Research Abstracts (ERA) (online database) <www.tandf.co.uk/era>*	2002
• *Family & Society Studies Worldwide <www.nisc.com>*	1997
• *FINDEX <www.publist.com>*	1999
• *FRANCIS. INIST/CNRS <www.inist.fr>*	1998
• *Guide to Social Science & Religion in Periodical Literature*	1997
• *Health Management Information Service (HELMIS)*	1997
• *IBZ International Bibliography of Periodical Literature <www.saur.de>*	2001
• *Index to Periodical Articles Related to Law*	1997

(continued)

- *"LABORDOC" Library-Periodicals Section "Abstracts Section"* 1996
- *National Library Database on Homelessness* 1997
- *OCLC Public Affairs Information Service <www.pais.org>*. 1998
- *Referativnyi Zhurnal (Abstracts Journal of the All-Russian Institute of Scientific and Technical Information–in Russian)*. 1997
- *Social Services Abstracts <www.csa.com>*. 1999
- *Social Work Abstracts <www.silverplatter.com/catalog/swab.htm>* 1997
- *Sociological Abstracts (SA) <www.csa.com>* 1997
- *Worldwide Political Science Abstracts (formerly: Political Science & Government Abstracts) <www.csa.com>* 1997

Special Bibliographic Notes related to special journal issues (separates) and indexing/abstracting:

- indexing/abstracting services in this list will also cover material in any "separate" that is co-published simultaneously with Haworth's special thematic journal issue or DocuSerial. Indexing/abstracting usually covers material at the article/chapter level.
- monographic co-editions are intended for either non-subscribers or libraries which intend to purchase a second copy for their circulating collections.
- monographic co-editions are reported to all jobbers/wholesalers/approval plans. The source journal is listed as the "series" to assist the prevention of duplicate purchasing in the same manner utilized for books-in-series.
- to facilitate user/access services all indexing/abstracting services are encouraged to utilize the co-indexing entry note indicated at the bottom of the first page of each article/chapter/contribution.
- this is intended to assist a library user of any reference tool (whether print, electronic, online, or CD-ROM) to locate the monographic version if the library has purchased this version but not a subscription to the source journal.
- individual articles/chapters in any Haworth publication are also available through the Haworth Document Delivery Service (HDDS).

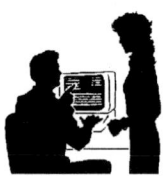

ABOUT THE EDITORS

Keith M. Kilty, PhD, is Professor in the College of Social Work at Ohio State University in Columbus and co-editor of the *Journal of Poverty*. He has published or presented more than 50 papers and is an editorial reviewer for *ALCOHOLISM: Clinical and Experimental Research*, the *Journal of Studies on Alcohol*, and the *American Education Research Journal*, and Assistant Editor for the *Journal of Drug Issues*. Dr. Kilty is a member of the Society for the Study of Social Problems and was Chair of the Poverty, Class, and Inequality Division. He is also Treasurer of the Bertha Capen Reynolds Society.

Elizabeth A. Segal, PhD, MSW, is Professor in the College of Social Work at Arizona State University in Tempe and co-editor of the *Journal of Poverty*. She has made many presentations and conducted workshops and seminars on various issues concerning social work and is the author of many articles, book chapters, book reviews, proceedings, and reports. She served as a policy analyst in Washington, DC as a Fellow of the American Association for the Advancement of Science. Dr. Segal is a member of the National Association of Social Workers, the Council on Social Work Education, and the Bertha Capen Reynolds Society.

ALL HAWORTH BOOKS AND JOURNALS ARE PRINTED ON CERTIFIED ACID-FREE PAPER

Rediscovering the Other America: The Continuing Crisis of Poverty and Inequality in the United States

CONTENTS

Rediscovering the Other America: The Continuing Crisis of Poverty and Inequality in the United States: Introduction   1
Keith M. Kilty
Elizabeth A. Segal

Fixing that Great Hodgepodge: Health Care for the Poor in the U.S.   7
Llewellyn J. Cornelius

Staying Poor in the Clinton Boom: Welfare Reform and the Nearby Labor Force   23
Frank Stricker

Political Promises for Welfare Reform   51
Elizabeth A. Segal
Keith M. Kilty

The "Other America" After Welfare Reform: A View from the Nonprofit Sector   69
David Sommerfeld
Michael Reisch

Gender Differences in the Economic Well-Being of Nonaged Adults in the United States   97
Martha N. Ozawa
Hong-Sik Yoon

Central Appalachia–Still the *Other* America   123
   Susan Sarnoff

Welfare Policy, Welfare Participants, and CalWORKS
   Caseworkers: How Participants Are Informed
   of Supportive Services   141
   Elizabeth Bartle
   Gabriela Segura

Making Experience Count in Policy Creation:
   Lessons from Appalachian Kentucky   163
   Christiana Miewald

THOUGHTS ON POVERTY AND INEQUALITY

Driving Out of Poverty in Private Automobiles   183
   Lisa M. Brabo
   Peter H. Kilde
   Patrick Pesek-Herriges
   Thomas Quinn
   Inger Sanderud-Nordquist

Index   197

Rediscovering the Other America: The Continuing Crisis of Poverty and Inequality in the United States: Introduction

Keith M. Kilty
Elizabeth A. Segal

Poverty and inequality are nothing new or unique to the United States. Both were brought to the Americas by European invaders beginning in the late fifteenth century. Spurred by dismal economic conditions in Europe, early explorers crossed the Atlantic in search of new wealth. As European colonies became established throughout the Americas, those in power found themselves in need of a stable work force, and Europeans and Africans were pressed into indentured servitude–and ultimately slavery–since voluntary migrants to the American colonies were few and far between. Those at the top, whether in Europe or in the American colonies, benefited immensely, while those at the bottom, regardless of their origins, found themselves oppressed and exploited (Galeano, 1973; Takaki, 1998). This gap between rich and poor, which had its origins five centuries ago, continues not only to persist but also to threaten the democratic foundation of this country. Unfortunately, many people here–especially those in power–suffer from a historical amnesia about poverty.

Keith M. Kilty is Professor, College of Social Work, Ohio State University, 1947 College Road, Columbus, OH 43210.
Elizabeth A. Segal is Professor, School of Social Work, Arizona State University, Box 871802, Tempe, AZ 85287-1802.

[Haworth co-indexing entry note]: "Rediscovering the Other America: The Continuing Crisis of Poverty and Inequality in the United States: Introduction." Kilty, Keith M., and Elizabeth A. Segal. Co-published simultaneously in *Journal of Poverty* (The Haworth Press, Inc.) Vol. 7, No. 1/2, 2003, pp. 1-6; and: *Rediscovering the Other America: The Continuing Crisis of Poverty and Inequality in the United States* (ed: Keith M. Kilty, and Elizabeth A. Segal) The Haworth Press, Inc., 2003, pp. 1-6. Single or multiple copies of this article are available for a fee from The Haworth Document Delivery Service [1-800-HAWORTH, 9:00 a.m. - 5:00 p.m. (EST). E-mail address: docdelivery@haworthpress.com].

© 2003 by The Haworth Press, Inc. All rights reserved.

Forty years ago, the United States was the dominant industrialized nation in the world. Large portions of Europe and Asia had been devastated by the destruction of World War II, putting the U.S. into a position of dominance for the rest of the twentieth century. For many people, there was a sense that poverty and inequality had disappeared from the U.S., that the affluence experienced by some was in fact experienced by most if not all. Yet poverty and inequality were deeply entrenched in this country, as Michael Harrington (1962) documented in *The Other America*. He was not the only one aware of the problem, but his seminal work is often given credit for awakening a new sense of urgency about poverty and inequality. Of course, others were also writing about these matters, and grassroots efforts to organize the disaffected were ongoing in many communities as well as nationally through the civil rights movement that had been resurrected in the 1950s. The critical issue is that poverty and inequality had to be rediscovered then. The problems had not in reality gone away but simply disappeared from the public policy and media agenda–just as they have now in the early years of the twenty-first century. As a result, it has once again become necessary to rediscover these social problems.

Certainly, social conditions in 2002 are different in some ways from 1962. Four decades ago, there was no standardized method of counting the poor. Now the federal government establishes an annual poverty threshold, and we have 40 years of historical data on the level of poverty in the U.S. There are serious questions about the adequacy of official definitions of poverty, and the annual statistics published by the Census Bureau need to be treated cautiously. Poverty is still technically calculated in terms of the cost of food, under the assumption that one-third of a family's disposable income goes to food (Segal & Brzuzy, 1998). That definition probably is no longer accurate–if it ever was. Further, a different poverty threshold is used for determining poverty among the elderly than among the non-elderly, with the elderly threshold some 10% lower than the non-elderly threshold. As a result, poverty among the elderly is likely understated as well.

More critical is the effort by many public officials to argue that recent "welfare reform" legislation has led to reductions in poverty. In fact, as Kilty and Segal (2001), among others, have noted, recent reductions in poverty rates have barely returned to where they were in 1979 and are still well above the historical low of 11.1% in 1973. During an era of supposed prosperity, we still not have seen poverty as low as it was prior to the beginning of the Reagan-Bush Era. More than 32 million people live below the official poverty line. That number equals the total populations of Tennessee, Kansas, Michigan, Wisconsin, and New Jersey combined (U.S. Census Bureau, 2001). The War on Poverty programs, never adequately funded, still had profound impacts on poverty levels in this country, and the single most effective poverty reduction program continues to be public old-age pensions administered through the Social Security Administration. At least 40% more older people would fall below the poverty line without their social security benefits (Social Security Administration, 2001). Public programs, in other words, work and work well–contrary to the protestations of many public and business officials.

Most public discussions about the poor now focus not on poverty but instead on "welfare" or "public assistance." Poverty and welfare are two entirely different matters. For two decades now, though, concern about welfare has dominated the rhetoric about social welfare and social problems. Yet the poor have always been largely on their own in this vastly wealthy land. Even at the peak of the AFDC program, two-thirds of those who were officially poor received no public assistance (Karger & Stoesz, 2002). Furthermore, two-thirds of those who received assistance were dependent children of women eligible for AFDC. Perhaps the easiest way to see who benefits from social welfare policy in the U.S. is to look at tax policy (Barlett & Steele, 1994). In fact, the single largest housing assistance program is the mortgage interest deduction available to those who itemize their taxes, and over half of that total benefit goes to those with family incomes in excess of $100,000.

Why do we seem to hate the poor in America? Why do we want to put them out of our awareness? Recent public policy, such as the Personal Responsibility and Work Opportunity Reconciliation Act (PRWORA) of 1996, was remarkably mean-spirited. Is that what we are as a people? Are we primarily motivated by greed? Perhaps some in this country are, but that is not true of all–or probably even most. Harrington is an example of a publicly outspoken critic of how things are in this country, one voice among many heard throughout our history. Our goal with this volume is to help once again in the rediscovery of poverty and inequality. We are now on the threshold of a new century, and yet there are still far too many of our citizens struggling to survive. In the following pages, we will document the nature of these struggles.

One of the most critical concerns for the poor and near-poor, the "other Americans" of the early twenty-first century, is health care. Even many in the middle live with anxiety about adequate health care protection. Cornelius addresses this in his article, "Fixing that Great Hodgepodge," in which he discusses first why there has been a lack of commitment to the poor. He presents a series of prescriptions that can ensure adequate and quality health care for the poor, beginning with the need to separate health care coverage from having a job. Even in good economic times, not everyone will have a job, and joblessness becomes increasingly critical as bad times envelop us, as is currently happening.

In fact, it may well be the nature of the labor market that keeps many people poor, as Stricker argues in his paper. He challenges current measures of both the poverty rate and the unemployment rate and describes what he calls the "nearby labor force," where many of those forced off welfare are finding themselves. Part-time and contingency work grow, and finding adequate employment becomes more difficult with downturns in the economy. Much unemployment and underemployment are actually hidden because of the way in which the employment rate is officially defined. Without institutional changes, the other Americans will continue to be forced to fend for themselves, particularly now that public assistance is no longer an entitlement.

What is the official rhetoric about welfare and poverty? What are public officials willing to say, not behind closed doors, but in public forums? How does that connect to issues of class, gender, and race? That is the focus of Segal and Kilty, who use critical discourse analysis to examine all of the speeches delivered in person in the House of Representatives on July 31, 1996–immediately before the final vote on PRWORA took place. This provided an opportunity to look at the influence of power on the creation of public policy and the perpetuation of oppression for those at the bottom of the social hierarchy.

For two years now, President George W. Bush has promulgated his belief in the ability of the private sector to solve the problem of poverty as well as to break the so-called cycle of dependency for those on public assistance. Can, in fact, the private sector be as effective as the public, particularly in terms of potential resources? It was the Great Depression that first led to large-scale federal involvement in social welfare, because of the failure of the private sector and local and state governments. In their article, Sommerfeld and Reisch look at how the non-profit sector is dealing with the declining caseloads caused by welfare reform. Increasing demands are being made on private organizations, particularly for emergency food and shelter.

While poverty rates have fallen for the elderly, that is not true for all. Women are particularly vulnerable to poverty as they get older. Ozawa and Yoon examine gender differences among the non-aged in the U.S. During the recent past, they show that the gender gap has widened, particularly for women who are not married. For the "baby boom" generation, which is now approaching retirement age, that increasing gender gap is likely to make later life difficult for many women. In essence, they will find themselves "growing" into poverty.

One of the groups that Harrington described in detail was Appalachians–a group that is now largely forgotten. In 1965, the Appalachian Regional Commission was established, and efforts were made to develop the region. However, this was a broad area, encompassing thirteen states, and the bulk of federal funding went into highway construction. Sarnoff revisits this population group and describes the extent to which many of the characteristics found by Harrington in 1962 continue to exist in central Appalachia.

The political rhetoric surrounding welfare reform was that welfare recipients needed to learn responsibility and hold down jobs in order to "escape" from welfare dependency. Those receiving assistance must become employed. California's response to this new legislation was the California Work Opportunity and Responsibility to Kids Program (CalWORKS). Bartle and Segura look at provisions for domestic violence, substance abuse, and mental health services in this program and whether or not caseworkers are properly informing recipients about such programs. In general, it appears that many recipients are receiving inadequate information or being discouraged by their caseworkers from seeking necessary services.

As we have seen, there are many inaccuracies and myths about welfare recipients and other poor people. Miewald takes us to Appalachian Kentucky, where activists in local communities have tried to affect public images about poverty and the poor. She describes this process as "making experience count in policy creation." Public policy about welfare and public assistance cannot change for the better without taking into account the actual experiences of the poor, especially poor parents.

In the last paper, Brabo and her associates describe a pilot program focused on getting people to their jobs. Many people live in areas where there is limited public transportation, and yet they must have reliable transportation to and from work. In most rural areas and small towns and even medium-sized cities, the primary source of transportation is the private automobile. Yet safe and reliable cars are often beyond the means of the poor, including the working poor. The question then becomes finding a way to help people in acquiring adequate private transportation, including making adequate down payments and getting reasonable interest rates on loans. The West Central Wisconsin Community Action Agency (West CAP) has developed just such a program.

The papers in this volume were selected from those presented at a conference titled, "Rediscovering the Other America: A National Forum on

Poverty and Inequality," which was held on August 18, 2002, in Chicago, Illinois. In addition to the *Journal of Poverty*, this forum was co-sponsored by the Poverty, Class and Inequality Division of the Society for the Study of Social Problems; the Society for the Study of Social Problems (SSSP); Sociologists for Women in Society; the School of Social Work, Loyola University (Chicago); the College of Arts and Sciences, Georgia State University; the College of Social Work, Ohio State University; the Center for Urban Research and Learning, Loyola University (Chicago); the SSSP Conflict, Social Action, and Change Division; the SSSP Family Division; the SSSP Health, Health Policy and Health Services Division; the SSSP Labor Studies Division; the SSSP Law and Society Division; and the SSSP Sociology and Social Welfare Division. We are indebted to the support of all these organizations and all the fine contributions to the National Forum.

REFERENCES

Bartlett, D. L. & Steele, J. B. (1994). *America: Who really pays the taxes?* New York: Touchstone.
Galeano, E. (1973). *Open veins of Latin America*. New York: Monthly Review.
Harrington, M. (1962). *The other America*. New York: Collier.
Karger, H. J. & Stoesz, D. (2002). *American social welfare policy*. Boston: Allyn and Bacon.
Kilty, K. M. & Segal, E. A. (2001). Introduction: Examining the impact of "ending welfare as we know it." *Journal of Poverty*, 5 (2), 1-4.
Segal, E. A. & Brzuzy, S. (1998). *Social welfare policy, programs, and practice*. Itasca, IL: Peacock.
Social Security Administration. (2001). *Fast facts and figures about social security*. (SSA Publication No. 13-11785). Washington, DC: Social Security Administration.
Takaki, R. (1998). *Strangers from a distant shore: A history of Asian Americans*. (Rev. ed.). Boston: Little, Brown.
U.S. Census Bureau. (2001). Statistical abstract of the United States: 2001. Washington, DC: U.S. Department of Commerce.

Fixing that Great Hodgepodge: Health Care for the Poor in the U.S.

Llewellyn J. Cornelius

SUMMARY. Like many of the poverty-based initiatives that emanated from the 1960s, America's commitment to providing health care for the poor is inconsistent at best. This paper highlights the evolution of health care coverage for the poor during the last half of the 20th century. Documentation on health care coverage preceding 1965 indicates that our initial commitment to the poor focused on a segment of the poor–the aged, the blind, the disabled and needy families–while neglecting working-age adults. This set the stage for the development of the Medicaid program in 1965 and remains the core of the groups who are covered by Medicaid today. It is suggested that the only way to meet the health care needs of all of the disadvantaged is by scrapping the current private and public health insurance mechanisms in favor of a more global, nonemployment-based health insurance coverage for all Americans. *[Article copies available for a fee from The Haworth Document Delivery Service: 1-800-HAWORTH. E-mail address: <docdelivery@haworthpress.com> Website: <http://www.HaworthPress.com> © 2003 by The Haworth Press, Inc. All rights reserved.]*

Llewellyn J. Cornelius is Associate Professor, University of Maryland at Baltimore, School of Social Work.

Address correspondence to: Llewellyn J. Cornelius, 525 W. Redwood Street, Baltimore, MD 21201.

The information reported in this paper reflects the views of the author and no official endorsement by the University of Maryland at Baltimore, School of Social Work is intended or should be inferred.

[Haworth co-indexing entry note]: "Fixing that Great Hodgepodge: Health Care for the Poor in the U.S." Cornelius, Llewellyn J. Co-published simultaneously in *Journal of Poverty* (The Haworth Press, Inc.) Vol. 7, No. 1/2, 2003, pp. 7-21; and: *Rediscovering the Other America: The Continuing Crisis of Poverty and Inequality in the United States* (ed: Keith M. Kilty, and Elizabeth A. Segal) The Haworth Press, Inc., 2003, pp. 7-21. Single or multiple copies of this article are available for a fee from The Haworth Document Delivery Service [1-800-HAWORTH, 9:00 a.m. - 5:00 p.m. (EST). E-mail address: docdelivery@haworthpress.com].

KEYWORDS. Poverty, uninsured, Medicaid

In spite of the acknowledged woeful neglect of the poor as summarized in Michael Harrington's book, *The Other America*, we begin the new millennium no better off than in 1962 when the book was first published. It is argued that in the case of health care we are in this situation because America never committed to meeting the health care needs for all the poor in the first place. We only focused on caring for the "worthy" poor, rather than addressing the needs of all of the disadvantaged. As caretakers of the poor, America decided that only some of them–children, persons with disabilities, and the elderly–were worthy of federal/state supported health-care coverage. Meanwhile, working age adults were left with obtaining health care coverage through work or paying for health care out of their own pockets. The purpose of this paper is to summarize how this patchwork of commitment evolved and to suggest how can we make a more consistent commitment to the poor in the future.

GARBAGE IN, GARBAGE OUT: HEALTH CARE COVERAGE BEFORE THE WAR ON POVERTY

Our "commitment" to providing health care coverage for the poor began in the depression. Before the early 1930s there was no private or public insurance coverage for health care services. Americans had to pay out of pocket for health care services (Starr, 1982; Anderson, 1984). Between the early 1930s and the passage of the Kerr-Mills program in 1960, America's commitment to providing health care for the poor was limited to a few states providing vendor payments to hospitals and physicians for services delivered to the aged, the blind, the disabled, and needy families, the provision of charity care at faith-based institutions and the provision of uncompensated care at institutions built with federal funds from the Hill-Burton program (the Hospital Survey and Construction Act of 1947) (Stuart and Blair, 1971; Anderson, 1984). In 1960, the Social Security Act was amended to provide matching funds for states to pay physicians and hospitals for delivering medical care to the aged who were poor (U.S. Department of Health Education and Welfare, 1962; Marmor, 2000).

THE MEDICAID PROGRAM

The Medicaid program, Title XIX of the Social Security Act, represented an expansion of earlier public insurance programs for the aged, the blind, the disabled, and the medically needy (U.S. Department of Health Education and Welfare, 1975). The 1965 legislation tied the eligibility for Medicaid to enrollment in one of two cash assistance programs: Aid to Families with Dependent Children (AFDC), and Supplemental Security Income (SSI) (U.S. Department of Health Education and Welfare, 1977). These programs served portions of the poor who met eligibility requirements based on resources, assets, and other criteria. In addition to providing coverage for the enrollees in these two programs, Medicaid had the option of extending coverage to other poor persons as well as to the "medically needy" whose family income was above the poverty line. States were given both the option to participate and to decide which services to provide over and above set minimally required services (U.S. Department of Health Education and Welfare, 1975). Although Medicaid was meant to improve access to medical care for the poor, Starr explains that when the Medicaid program began in 1965, it "omitted from coverage most two-parent families, and childless couples, widows, and other single persons under the age of sixty-five years, families with fathers working at low paying jobs, and the medically needy in twenty-two states that did not provide coverage" (Starr, 1982, 374).

The federal government did not have direct control over the Medicaid program as a whole, since the role of implementing the program was left to the states. Considerable diversity in the range and extent of covered services evolved. One state (Arizona) did not develop a Medicaid-type program until the 1980s. Thus, even from its inception, the Medicaid program did not cover all persons who live in poverty. Although there have been several expansions to the program since 1965, these gaps in coverage of the poor continue today.

A comparison of Medicaid, AFDC, and SSI program enrollment data during the period of 1974 through 1996 highlights the mismatch between the estimates of the number of Americans living in poverty and the number of persons covered by Medicaid (Table 1). In 1974 over 23 million Americans lived in poverty. At the same time, Medicaid provided health insurance coverage to 20.8 million Americans. If one assumes, based on program eligibility criteria, that Medicaid covered all of the SSI (4 million) and the AFDC recipients (10.9 million), that still left nearly 10 million poor Americans without health insurance (Table 1). Similarly, in 1986 there were 32.7 million Americans living in poverty. Of this popu-

TABLE 1. Numbers of Recipients of Medicaid, SSI or AFDC (in Thousands), United States, 1974-1995

Characteristics	1974	1978	1986	1995
Number of Persons in Poverty[a]				
Under 18 years of age	10,156	9,931	12,876	14,665
18-64 years	10,132	11,332	16,017	18,442
65 and older	3,085	3,233	3,477	3,318
Total	23,273	24,496	32,370	36,525
Number of Medicaid Recipients[b]				
Aged	3,805	4,429	3,140	4,119
Blind	136	131	82	92
Disabled	2,280	3,109	4,000	5,767
Children under 21	10,110	11,626	10,031	17,164
Adults in families with dependent children	4,511	5,705	5,647	7,603
Total	20,842	25,000	22,518	36,282
Number of SSI Recipients[c]				
Aged	2,286	1,968	1,473	1,446
Blind	75	77	83	84
Disabled	1,636	2,172	2,713	4,984
Total	3,996	4,217	4,269	6,514
Average Monthly AFDC Caseload[d]				
Children	7,821	7,220	7,165	9,275
All recipients	10,960	10,497	10,813	13,169

Sources: [a] U.S. Census Bureau (2000). *Current Population Reports: Poverty in the United States, 1999,* Table B-2; [b] U.S. Department of Health Education and Welfare, Health Care Financing Administration (1977). *Data on the Medicaid Program: Eligibility, services, expenditures, fiscal years 1966-1977* – Table 13, U.S. Department of Health and Human Services, Health Care Financing Administration (1990). *Health Care Financing Program Statistics; Medicare and Medicaid Data Book* 1990–Table 4.12, U.S. Department of Health and Human Services, Health Care Financing Administration (1996). *Medicaid Statistics: Program and Financial Statistics Fiscal Year 1995*–Table 2; [c] Committee on Ways and Means, U.S. House of Representatives (1996). *1996 Green Book: Background material and data on programs within the jurisdiction of the committee on ways and means*–Table 4.1; [d] Committee on Ways and Means, U.S. House of Representatives (1996). *1996 Green Book: Background material and data on programs within the jurisdiction of the committee on ways and means*–Table 8.1.

lation, 4.3 million received SSI and 10.8 million received AFDC. This left a potential 17.6 million who fell through the cracks as they did not meet the mandatory eligibility criteria for Medicaid. While these numbers do not directly communicate the numbers of poor uninsured Americans, it has been reported that between 1980 and 1992 the Medicaid program consistently enrolled only a small portion of young working-age males or persons who were between 45 and 64 years of age (Health Care Financing Review, 1995).

Previously, comparisons were made of the numbers of persons who were enrolled in Medicaid between 1974 and 1986. Data from the 1995 program year reveals that there was a growth in the number of children enrolled in Medicaid (Table 1). There were almost twice as many children covered by Medicaid in 1995 as in 1974 (17.1 million versus 10.1 million). Kamerman (1996) suggests that some of the expansion in coverage in the early 1990s can be attributed to Medicaid picking up the slack when employers downsized medical coverage or dropped dependent coverage. Holahan, Weiner and Wallin (1998) suggest that some of the expansion in coverage during the same period can be attributed to the federally imposed eligibility expansions for children and pregnant women as well as to changes in the SSI eligibility rules for children. However, in spite of the expansion in the number of poor children covered by Medicaid after 1986, it was estimated that in 1996 as many as 40 percent of the children who were eligible for Medicaid were not enrolled in the program (Kenney, Haley and Ullman, 1999).

While the program data provides an indirect view of the gaps in coverage for the poor, data from the National Health Interview Survey conducted by the National Center for Health Statistics (Table 2) provide a more direct estimate of the gaps in insurance coverage for the poor. Data on health insurance coverage for the poor by age during the period of 1984 through 1999 reveal three scenarios: a consistent commitment to the elderly who are poor; a growth in coverage for poor children; and a consistent lack of coverage for poor adults between the ages of 18 and 64 (Table 2). Between 1984 and 1999 the percent of poor children (under 18) who were covered by Medicaid increased from 43.1 percent to 59.9 percent, while the percent who had private insurance declined (from 23.2 to 16.7 percent). The increase in the number of children on Medicaid offset the decline in the number with private insurance, thus the percent of uninsured children dropped from 28.9 percent to 21.6 percent over this 16-year time period (Table 2). Over the same period, around 40 percent of poor adults (ages 18 to 64) were uninsured. The rate of uninsured adults ages 18 to 64 increased from 39.2 percent in 1984 to 43.7 percent in 1999 (Table 2). Finally, all poor persons over 65 had some health insurance during this period (Table 2).

WHAT ACCOUNTS FOR THE LACK OF COMMITMENT TO THE POOR?

It was suggested earlier that changes in the economy and federal responses to these changes led to increases in the number of persons covered by Medicaid. In addition to these factors, America's degree of

TABLE 2. Insurance Status of Persons Living in Poverty, by Age, United States, 1984-1999

Characteristics	1984	1989	1994	1999
Percent of persons under 18[a]				
With private insurance	23.2	17.5	12.3	16.7
With Medicaid	43.1	47.8	64.3	59.9
Without health insurance	28.9	31.6	22.1	21.6
Percent of persons ages 18-64[a,b]				
With private insurance	36.4	31.7	28.5	30.9
With Medicaid	20.5	25.2	25.4	20.7
Without health insurance	39.2	39.4	41.9	43.7
Percent of persons aged 65 and older[a]				
With private insurance and Medicare	43.4	46.1	43.6	28.3
With Medicaid and Medicare	27.6	28.2	33.4	35.7
With Medicare only	27.9	26.4	23.6	28.4

[a] Percents may not add to 100 due to rounding error.

[b] Percents for the 18-64 population were computed using the population counts of the persons in poverty from the current population reports and the data provided from Tables 128-130 of Health United States, 2001.

Sources: U.S. Department of Health and Human Services, Centers for Disease Control, National Center for Health Statistics. *Health United States, 2001*–Tables 128-130 and U.S. Census Bureau (2000). *Current Population Reports: Poverty In the United States, 1999*, Table B-2.

commitment to providing health care coverage to the poor was influenced by responses to concerns about the costs of medical care, attempts to modify America's cash assistance program for the poor, and responses to political pressures to develop a national health insurance plan. Earlier, it was indicated that the federal government did not have control over the costs of administering the Medicaid program, because it was a joint federal/state program. Between 1965 and 1984, the federal share of health care expenditures tripled from 10.1 percent to 29.6 percent (National Center for Health Statistics, 1985). As the federal share of the Medicaid program started to spiral upward, the government implemented several cost-cutting mechanisms. The first cost-cutting plan called for the reduction of the federal commitment to Medicaid funding by 3 percent in fiscal year 1982, 4 percent in 1983 and 4.5 percent in 1984 (Altman, 1983) and were included in the Omnibus Budget Reconciliation Act of 1981. Further reductions were anticipated along with the expectation that the states would have to decide how much of the burden for Medicaid they would begin to assume, given successive federal reductions over the next five years (Health Care Financial Management, 1986).

A second cost-cutting tactic was the movement of Medicaid patients into managed-care programs, where the providers would receive a fixed fee for providing care to their patients. The free choice of provider requirement for the Medicaid program was waived, enabling states to develop innovative arrangements for enrolling Medicaid-eligibles with preferred providers or case-management oriented primary care networks and by prescribing the amount which Medicaid recipients would pay out-of-pocket for certain optional, as well as mandatory, services (Altman, 1983; Mundinger, 1985).

A third cost-cutting tactic was to decrease or freeze the reimbursements to physicians who cared for Medicaid patients. Reimbursement fees for services provided to Medicaid patients have been traditionally much lower than for services provided to other patients (Norton, 1999; U.S. General Accounting Office, 2001a). This gap in fees has contributed to the reluctance of some physicians to accept Medicaid patients (Gabel and Rice, 1985; Norton, 1999). The impact of these various cost-cutting arrangements has been a decrease in the amount of medical care received by disadvantaged people (Davis and Rowland, 1983) and an increase in the percent of persons who delayed seeking medical treatment because they can not afford it (Aday et al., 1984).

In response to concerns about the effect of cost containment on the quality of health care, policymakers attempted to expand health insurance coverage for both poor and non-poor uninsured Americans. The mechanism that was used for expanding this coverage was the formulation of a national health insurance plan for all Americans. While several proposals were formulated, the most notable plan was the Clinton plan (the Health Security Act) which was first introduced as H.R 3600 (103rd Congress). The central idea was that Americans would be covered under one health plan, both the employed and unemployed, young and old, rich and poor alike. If enacted, it would have minimized the problem of inconsistent health care coverage of the poor as they would have been treated the same way as other Americans.

However, the Clinton plan and its derivatives failed because of several obstacles. These obstacles included: opposition from health providers and institutions; a lack of consensus among businesses; a lack of consensus among elected officials regarding the plan; and the inability of consumers to understand the complexity of the plan. With regards to health care providers, members of the American Medical Association and other health providers were opposed to the plan because they perceived that the consumer had fewer choices for selecting providers, or physicians would have to ration the care they provided under the plan (Hogeboom, 1994; Gibbs and Aunapu, 1993). Small businesses were opposed to the plan because they did not like the mandatory participation requirement (Franklin, 1995). In one case, lobbyists for small businesses pressured members of the 44-member House Energy and Commerce Committee (one of the committees that reviewed the Clinton plan) into voting against the Clinton plan. As a result of this political pressure, the bill never made it out of this committee. All 17 of the Republican Party members opposed the bill and only 22 of the 27 Democrats supported the bill (Franklin, 1995).

While none of the various national health insurance proposals was adopted, one of the outcomes of this push for national health insurance was the avocation for the extension of Medicaid coverage to all poor children (Dentzer, 1996). This laid the groundwork for the passage of the Children Health Insurance Program, a health insurance program for children who lived in families with incomes up to 200 percent of the poverty line.

No sooner was the Clinton plan defeated than another policy rolled through Congress that affected the delivery of health care to the poor: the welfare reform legislation. Concurrent with the action that was taking place on the Clinton plan, members of Congress were developing legislation to replace the AFDC program with a more temporary cash assistance program called Temporary Assistance to Needy Families (TANF). One of the issues that needed to be addressed in this activity was how to handle the relationship between Medicaid and AFDC, since historically Medicaid eligibility was tied to enrollment in AFDC or SSI. Thus people who lost AFDC or SSI typically found themselves without health insurance coverage. While there were attempts in the 1980s to implicitly break the ties between AFDC or SSI and Medicaid (Tanenbaum, 1995; Kamerman, 1998), the link was explicitly broken when the Personal Responsibility and Work Opportunity Reconciliation Act (PRWORA) was passed in 1996 (Ku and Coughlin, 1997).

In theory, this should have led to an increase in Medicaid coverage for the poor. However, even after the passage of the PRWORA act, otherwise qualified needy individuals were hindered from submitting applications for Medicaid (Chavkin, Romero and Wise, 2000; Mann and Schott, 1999; Ellwood, 1999) because the same form was used for their TANF application and their Medicaid application. The failure to correct this problem led to a drop in the Medicaid caseload and an increase in the number of uninsured ex-welfare recipients (Ku and Garrett, 2000). Thus, according to the National Survey of American Families:

> only slightly over half of the women who leave welfare are still on Medicaid or other state health insurance in the first six months after leaving, and one third have no health insurance at all. By the time they have been off of welfare for a year or more, less than one quarter of these women are receiving Medicaid benefits and about half are without health insurance. (Garrett and Holahan, 2000, p. 1)

In short, because some public agencies did not aggressively communicate this policy change to the indigent, some persons were dropped from Medicaid, even though they still qualified for care.

This bungle was also complicated by the concurrent passage of a more liberal health insurance program for poor children entitled the Children Health Insurance Program (CHIP). CHIP was designed to bridge the gap in coverage for poor children. In order to facilitate enrollment in CHIP, the program simplified the enrollment requirements. At the same time, the CHIP program provided higher physician reimbursement rates than Medicaid (U.S. General Accounting Office, 2000), which had increased provider participation in the program. However, the CHIP program, like Medicaid, had its own hurdles. One study reported that 53 percent of all low income parents did not even know their state had a child health insurance program and 44 percent did not understand that they did not have to be on welfare for their child to enroll in this program (Kenney, Haley and Dubay, 2001). In the end, the legacy of the failure to adopt a national health insurance plan in the middle of the 1990s was a return to the status quo. The poor had to contend with programs that created hurdles and obstacles, rather than opening doors for them.

WHAT CAN BE DONE FOR THE POOR?

How do we bridge the gap in insurance coverage for the poor? We need to revisit the last round of national health insurance policy options, and improve on what has been developed. It was stated earlier that the Clinton plan ran into several obstacles: a lack of understanding from average citizens regarding what the plan meant; providers' feeling that consumers would not have a choice of plans and options for coverage, and employers' feeling that they were required to participate in this venture. In order to address these problems, I suggest that we advocate for the development of a comprehensive, across-the-board health insurance plan that addresses these issues, with an eye towards developing a broad based plan that is universal in scope, yet flexible in coverage. As such I would suggest the following changes to the way in which we provide health insurance in the United States.

- *Break the tie between having a job and having health insurance.* Under the current system most health insurance coverage is employment-based, but the chances you are covered vary by the size of the company you work for. Nearly one-third of the workforce works in companies with fewer than 50 employees, yet only 36 percent of employers with fewer than 10 employees provided health insurance, compared with 71 percent of the companies that employ between 10 and 49 persons, and 96 percent of the companies that had 50 employees or more (U.S. General Accounting Office, 2001b). The reason for this is that it is more expensive for small companies than for large companies to provide coverage for their employees (United States General Accounting Office 2001b). By removing the link between employment and health care coverage, we open the door for the development of a plan that would not be marginalized and stigmatized. It is well known that social policies that are broad based (employment-based health care coverage, unemployment insurance, Medicare, Social Security) are viewed more favorably than those that serve only a margin of the population (Medicaid, TANF, etc.). One could break the tie between insurance and employment by eliminating the need to have a job as the only mechanism for collecting what would become the individual contribution to the health insurance plan (like a payroll deduction for federal income tax similar to what was suggested in the American Health Security Act plan sponsored by Representative McDermutt and Senator Wellstone [Dentzer, 1994]). Thus, like a federal income tax, all persons in a certain age group (e.g., between the ages of 18 and 70) pay the costs of the contribution to an individual or family health insurance plan. Like the collection of the federal income tax, the workplace serves only as a convenient collection point for these funds. In the same manner as the collection of the federal income tax, one can elect not to pay their share of the costs of the plan at their place of employment and instead pay for their share of the costs of the plan when they file their annual income tax. In fact, this financing arrangement is similar to what usually happens in the workplace for those who have employment-sponsored private insurance: The individual pays a portion of the cost as a payroll deduction, while the company pays the majority of the cost as a "fringe benefit." Under this new plan, individuals would be expected to pay a modest percent (e.g., 25 percent) of the annual premium for the plan as a payroll deduction, while the remaining 75 percent would come from implementing a valued added tax (VAT). As indicated by Cornelius (2000) and Rifkin (1995), a VAT is a tax on nonessential goods and services. Thus, it is a tax on everything but food, clothing, shelter, housing and medical care. Fifty-nine countries outside of the U.S. administer a VAT tax. The difference between the proposed and the current option is that employers usually pay a large portion of the annual premium as a "fringe benefit" to the employer, while the employee pays a portion out of his or her pocket as a payroll deduction. This move would shift the majority of the cost from the employer to society as a whole.

- *Develop community alliances as a mechanism for lowering the costs of health insurance premiums.* The second piece to the plan, which is just as important as separating health insurance from employment, is fostering the types of community alliances needed to balance the costs of coverage across large numbers of people. This option was included in the Clinton plan, but not other plans (Dentzer, 1994). Rather than being pooled together by the size of the company (the current scenario in America) pools of individuals are collected geographically for the purposes of estimating the costs of health insurance premiums. This pooling together of individuals would address the problems individuals encounter when they attempt to buy health insurance alone or small companies encounter when they attempt to purchase health insurance for their employees.
- *Provide an insurance tax credit for the poor.* Next, we need to acknowledge that the poor may need some type of "tax credit" to absorb some of the cost of the individual portion of the premiums. This would make it more affordable for the poor to participate in the plan.
- *Make the plan easy to understand and involve coalitions in the process.* Given that the Clinton plan was over 1,300 pages long, we need to do a better job of communicating the basics of the plan and to make participating in the plan meaningful for all. As such, community coalitions should be involved in the formulation and dissemination of the information regarding the plan. They should also be involved in the assessment of the protection of patient rights under the plan. We need to be able to summarize the basic elements of the plan. (It should address the following questions: What does it cost

individuals and families? What does it cover? How does one enroll in the plan? How does one select or change providers under the plan? What are their consumer rights?) This document needs to be written in nontechnical language that a person with a sixth- or seventh-grade reading level can understand. It should be disseminated in written and other formats to accommodate persons who cannot read, hear, or see. It should be multilingual to accommodate persons whose primary language is not English. Simplifying the plan and developing coalitions to support the plan increase the chance that citizens would be able to galvanize support for the adoption and implementation of such a plan.

- *Factor into the plan administrative costs for allowing for consumer choice in the selection of one of several provider options under the same cost scenario.* This is needed to address the providers' concerns about the lack of consumer choice options under the Clinton plan.
- *Work with providers to develop a minimum set of covered services.* Since providers will be expected to render services under this plan, it would be important to have them develop a minimum set of covered services under the plan, based on the expected costs of the plan. In addition, they would be expected to develop options for supplemental coverage for those who want elective services that are not covered by such a plan. In addition to having providers develop the plan, it will be necessary to provide consumer oversight over the implementation of the plan, so as to keep the local, state and federal bureaucracy accountable regarding their commitment to the disadvantaged. In this case, consumer oversight means community-based nonprofessional/non-health care providers. The rationale is its importance to empower the local community to monitor the administration of such a plan (especially given the potential large sources of revenue that would be at stake).

These recommendations are offered because it is believed that the needs of the disadvantaged will not be met simply be modifying a program that is already inadequate, i.e., Medicaid. Medicaid carries with it administrative hurdles and inadequate financial incentives for provider participation. Thus, any attempt to expand coverage to the poor using this mechanism would only lead to the poor being treated like second-class citizens. On the other hand, it is suggested here that we will never fairly address the health care needs of the "other America" unless we link them to our plight. By scrapping the private health insurance and Medicare plan and developing a uniform national health insurance plan, the poor and the non-poor tie their fates and successes to each other.

REFERENCES

Aday, L.A. et al. (1984). *Access to Medical Care in the U.S.: Who Has It, Who Doesn't.* Chicago: Pluribus Press, Inc.

Altman, D. (1983) Health Care for the Poor. *Annals of the American Academy of Political and Social Sciences, 468:* 103-121.

Anderson, O.W. (1984). Health Services in the United States: A Growth Enterprise for a Hundred Years. In T. J. Litman and L. S. Robins (eds), *Health Politics and Policy.* New York: John Wiley and Sons.

Chavkin, W., Romero, D., & Wise, P.H. (2000). State welfare reform politics and declines in health insurance. *American Journal of Public Health, 90*: 900-908.

Committee on Ways and Means, U.S. House of Representatives (1996). *1996 Green Book: Background material and data on programs within the jurisdiction of the committee on ways and means.* Washington, DC: U.S. Government Printing Office.

Cornelius, L.J. (2000). Financial Barriers to Health Care for Latinos: Poverty and Beyond. *Journal of Poverty: Innovations on social, political and economic inequalities* Vol. 4, #1 2000, 4 (1/2): 63-83 and in *Latino Poverty in the New Century: Inequalities, Challenges and Barriers* Edited by Maria Vidal de Haymes, PhD, Keith M. Kilty, PhD, and Elizabeth A. Segal, Binghamton, NY: Haworth Press.

Davis, K., & Rowland, D. (1983) Uninsured and Underserved: Inequities in Health Care in the United States. *Milbank Memorial Fund Quarterly, 61*: 149-176.

Dentzer, S. (1994). Sizing up the other plans. *U.S. News and World Report, 116*: 30-34.

Dentzer, S. (1996). For mercy's sake, let's cover the kids. *U.S. News & World Report,* 121: 69.

Ellwood, M. (1999). *The Medicaid Eligibility Maze: Coverage expands, but enrollment problems persist. Findings from a five state study.* Washington, DC: The Urban Institute.

Franklin, D. (1995). Tommy Boggs and the death of health care reform. *Washington Monthly, 27*: 31-38.

Gabel J.R., & Rice, T. H. (1985). Reducing Public Expenditures for Physicians: The Price of Paying Less. *Journal of Health Politics, Policy and Law, 9*: 595-609.

Garrett, B., & Holahan, J. (2000). *Welfare leavers, Medicaid coverage and private health insurance.* Washington, DC: The Urban Institute.

Gibbs, N., & Aunapu, G. (1993). Here comes doctor no. *Time, 142*: 26-29.

Harrington, M. (1962). *The other America.* New York, New York: Macmillan Health Care Financial Management (1986). 40: 5-7.

Hogeboom, W.L. (1994). Medical progress. *Commonweal, 121*: 7.

Holahan, J., Wiener, J., & Wallin, S. (1998). *Health policy for the low income population: Major findings from the assessing the New Federalism Case Studies.* Washington, DC: The Urban Institute.

Kamerman, S.B. (1996). The new politics of child and family policies. *Social Work, 41*: 453-465.

Kenney, G., Haley, J., & Dubay, L. (2001). *How familiar are low-income parents with Medicaid and SCHIP?* Washington, DC: The Urban Institute.

Kenney, G.M., Haley, J.M., & Ullman, F. (1999). *Most uninsured children are in families served by government programs.* Washington, DC: The Urban Institute.

Ku, L., & Coughlin, T.A. (1997). *How the new welfare reform law affects Medicaid.* Washington, DC: The Urban Institute.

Ku, L., & Garrett, B. (2000). *How welfare reform and economic factors affect Medicaid participation: 1984-96.* Washington, DC: The Urban Institute.

Mann, C., & Schott, L. (1999). Ensuring that eligible families receive Medicaid when cash assistance is denied or terminated. *Policy and practice of public human services, 57*: 6-10.

Marmor, T.R. (2000). *The Politics of Medicare (Second Edition).* Hawthorne, NY: Aldine De Gruyter.

Mundinger, M. O. (1985) Health Service Funding Cuts and the Declining Health of the Poor. *New England Journal of Medicine, 313*: 44-46.

Norton, S. (1999). *Recent trends in Medicaid Physician Fees, 1993-1998.* Washington, DC: The Urban Institute.

Rifkin, J. (1995). *The end of work: The decline of the global labor force and the dawn of the post market era.* New York: G. Putnam's Sons.

Starr, P. (1982) *The Social Transformation of American Medicine: The Rise of a Sovereign Professional and the Making of a Vast Industry.* New York: Basic Books Incorporated.

Stuart, B. C., & Blair, L.A. (1971). *Health care and income: The distributional impacts of Medicaid and Medicare Nationally and in the state of Michigan. (Second edition).* Lansing, MI: State of Michigan, Department of Social Services.

Tanenebaum, S.J. (1995). Medicaid eligibility policy in the 1980s: Medical utilitarianism and the "deserving" poor. *Journal of Health Politics, Policy and Law, 20*: 933-954.

U.S. Census Bureau (2000). *Current Population Reports: Poverty in the United States, 1999,* Washington, DC: U.S. Government Printing Office.

U.S. Department of Health, Education and Welfare (1962). Health Insurance for Aged Person. Report submitted to the committee on ways and means, House of Representatives by the secretary of health, education and welfare, July 24, 1961. in U.S. Department of Health Education and Welfare (ed). *Background on Medicare 1957-1962. Volume 12 85th-87th Congress. Reports, studies and congressional considerations on health legislation.* Washington, DC: Department of Health, Education and Welfare, Social Security Administration.

U.S. Department of Health, Education and Welfare (1975). History and evolution of Medicaid. In Spiegel, A.D., Podair, S. (eds). *Medicaid: Lessons for National Health Insurance.* Rockville, MD: Aspen Systems Corporation.

U.S. Department of Health Education and Welfare, Health Care Financing Administration (1977). *Data on the Medicaid Program: Eligibility, services, expenditures, fiscal years 1966-1977.* Washington, DC: U.S. Government Printing Office.

U.S. Department of Health and Human Services, (2001) Centers for Disease Control, National Center for Health Statistics. *Health United States, 2001.* Retrieved January 26, 2002 from http://www.cdc.gov/nchs/products/pubs/pubd/hus/hus.htm

U.S. Department of Health and Human Services, (1985) Centers for Disease Control, National Center for Health Statistics. *Health, United States, 1985.* DHHS Publication No. (PHS) 85-1232. Washington, DC: U.S. Government Printing Office.

U.S. Department of Health and Human Services, Health Care Financing Administration (1990). *Health Care Financing Program Statistics; Medicare and Medicaid Data Book 1990* Woodlawn, MD: Health Care Financing Administration.

U.S. Department of Health and Human Services, Health Care Financing Administration (1996). *Medicaid Statistics: Program and Financial Statistics Fiscal Year 1995.* Woodlawn, MD: Health Care Financing Administration.

U.S. General Accounting Office (2001a). *Medicaid and SCHIP: States' Enrollment and Payment Policies Can Affect Children's Access to Care.* Washington, DC: U.S. Government Printing Office.

U.S. General Accounting Office (2001b). *Private Health Insurance: Small Employers Continue to Face Challenges in Providing Coverage.* Washington, DC: U.S. Government Printing Office.

U.S. General Accounting Office (2000). *Medicaid and SCHIP: Comparisons of Outreach, Enrollment Practices, and Benefit.* Washington, DC: U.S. Government Printing Office.

Staying Poor in the Clinton Boom: Welfare Reform and the Nearby Labor Force

Frank Stricker

SUMMARY. Much poverty for employable Americans is caused not by welfare dependence or lack of schooling and skills, but by a labor glut that keeps many Americans unemployed or underemployed, and suppresses wage levels. In the 1980s and '90s employers slashed their workforces and the Federal Reserve Board often restrained economic growth to keep prices and wages from climbing too rapidly. Meanwhile, welfare reform cured little poverty and added millions to an already flooded labor pool. While it is well known that highly publicized monthly unemployment rates underestimate real joblessness, this article highlights previously ignored populations. It suggests that there is an iron law that American leaders resist growth that would eliminate unemployment and push official poverty rates below the 11% levels reached in the 1970s and the year 2000. It follows that to solve poverty there must be institutional changes–high minimum wages, union organization, more in-

---

Frank Stricker is Professor of History at California State University, Dominguez Hills, Carson, CA 90747 (E-mail: frnkstricker@aol.com).

The author thanks Deborah Schopp, Tom Larsen, Linda Pomerantz, students in the 2002 poverty class, and the Los Angeles Social History Research Seminar for their suggestions, and Alexis Schopp for aid in composing the figures.

The author benefited from a summer grant from the office of Vice-President Donald Castro, CSUDH.

[Haworth co-indexing entry note]: "Staying Poor in the Clinton Boom: Welfare Reform and the Nearby Labor Force." Stricker, Frank. Co-published simultaneously in *Journal of Poverty* (The Haworth Press, Inc.) Vol. 7, No. 1/2, 2003, pp. 23-49; and: *Rediscovering the Other America: The Continuing Crisis of Poverty and Inequality in the United States* (ed: Keith M. Kilty, and Elizabeth A. Segal) The Haworth Press, Inc., 2003, pp. 23-49. Single or multiple copies of this article are available for a fee from The Haworth Document Delivery Service [1-800-HAWORTH, 9:00 a.m. - 5:00 p.m. (EST). E-mail address: docdelivery@haworthpress.com].

© 2003 by The Haworth Press, Inc. All rights reserved.

come supports, and, perhaps, real government jobs. And that means a new politics. *[Article copies available for a fee from The Haworth Document Delivery Service: 1-800-HAWORTH. E-mail address: <docdelivery@haworthpress.com> Website: <http://www.HaworthPress.com> © 2003 by The Haworth Press, Inc. All rights reserved.]*

KEYWORDS. Unemployment, Nearby Labor Force, Bill Clinton, welfare reform

INTRODUCTION

Why, forty years after *The Other America* and the War on Poverty, does the United States still have 30 million poor people? Why, at the end of the longest economic boom in American history, was the poverty rate still over 11% and the near-poverty rate at least another 10%? Why does the United States usually have the highest poverty rate among the rich nations? In part, I will argue, because the American economy generates poverty and severe income inequality, and because the conservatism of American politics and policy means that not enough is done to counteract these normal economic outcomes. This paper is a memorial to Michael Harrington's pioneering work, but it is also an effort to understand poverty not as an other America but as an extreme reflection of the forces that make for hardship in the lives of millions of non-poor Americans. This paper puts unemployment and class at the center of poverty studies. Harrington would understand.

The United States has always been rather a laggard in protecting its citizens from the ravages of the marketplace, but in the 1970s, the forces of extreme conservatism gained extra momentum. The call to "get a job," long the cry of opponents of welfare, gained new power. Anti-welfare sentiment in Washington reached one peak in the Reagan years and another in 1996 with the repeal of AFDC.

The '90s were unusual in that two main conservative-centrist solutions to poverty were put to the test. The first was ending the entitlement to welfare benefits; the second was a booming economy. Both conservatives and liberals had long believed that growth was an effective and painless method for solving poverty. Moreover, welfare reform depended on growth to supply jobs for those ejected from the rolls. In many ways, welfare reform and growth were ideological twins, both emphasizing that work, not government income, job, and training programs, was the cure for poverty.

What was the outcome of economic expansion and welfare shrinkage in the '90s? The continuation of extreme income inequalities and lower but still high poverty rates. While stock market values increased many times during the decade, low-income Americans did not fare so well. They took on mountains of debt to maintain consumption; the net worth of the poorest 40% of the households fell 80% (Walsh, 2000; Collins, Leondar-Wright, and Sklar, 1999, p. 7). The welfare rolls declined sharply but most who left welfare stayed poor. Poverty rates did not decline as much as one would have expected in a booming economy. They fell from 15.1% (1993) to 11.3% in 2000, a welcome contrast to the '80s, but no lower than the 1970s (Figure 1).

Things were even worse than poverty rates indicated. About 22% of all American children under six lived in poor households in 1997, more than in 1979 (18.1%). Also, people who were poor in the late 1990s were poorer; only 30% of them fell below *half* the poverty line in 1975, but

FIGURE 1. U.S. Poverty Rates, 1960-2000

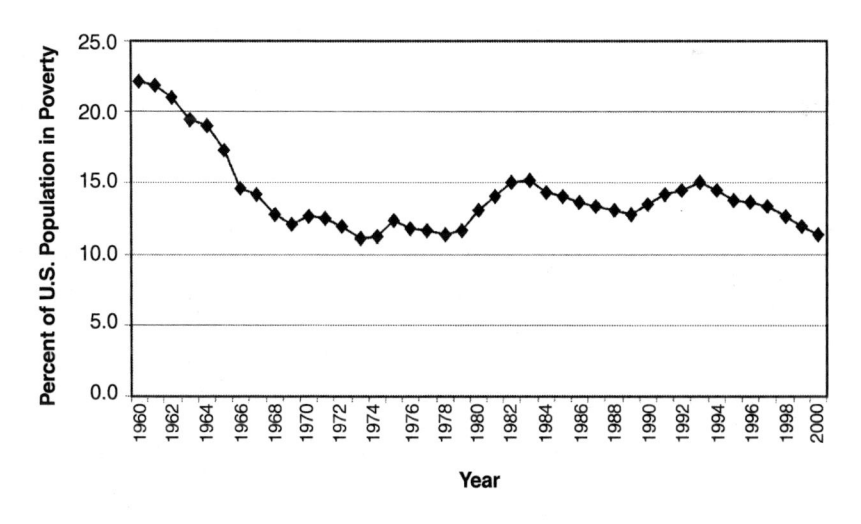

Source: U.S. Bureau of Census (2001, p.18)

41% did in 1997 (Mishel, Bernstein, and Schmitt, 1999, p. 291). These figures are even more shocking when we recall that they were based on one half of the already low federal poverty threshold of $17,000 for a family of four. It was ludicrous to think that a family paying $6000 to $10,000 a year for housing but with $18,000 total annual income was not poor. A poverty line raised to $21,000 would have been a modest improvement. Even that small increase yielded 46,000,000 people, or 17% of all Americans and 40% of all young children in poverty in the late '90s (Newton, 2000, pp. 1, 7; U.S. Bureau of the Census, 2001; Magnum, Sum, and Fogg, 2000). These large numbers of poor and near poor Americans were the harvest of a decade of economic growth and welfare reform.

Why did the long economic boom and radical welfare reform not produce better results? What happened to people who left welfare? Why did economic growth not lift Americans out of poverty as efficiently as it had in the 1940s, 1950s, and 1960s? The answer to these questions is the subject of this paper. I reject two common views that focus on the defects of poor people. Some claim that the poor lack skills; more on that later. Others assert that the poor are warped by underclass values that reward crime, laziness, and welfare dependence. But the underclass theory explains only a tiny fraction of the poverty population (Murray, 1999, pp. 12-15; Auletta, 1983, pp. 27-30; Ricketts and Sawhill, 1988). Contrary to much that was heard in the '90s, I believe that the root of job-related poverty is not that poor people lack modern skills or good attitudes, but rather that, first, there aren't enough jobs that pay a living wage; second, that a glut of workers keeps wages down; and third, that the American political process allows too many of the benefits of growth to go to the rich.

Much of this paper focuses on labor markets, which have tilted ever more in employers' favor. Three areas have been especially important: thirty years of deindustrialization, plant closures, and corporate and government policies that exacerbated employee insecurity; the weakening of unions and minimum wage laws that offset market-generated poverty; and, finally, a huge reservoir of workers that keeps wages down.

The unemployment point is the economic foundation of everything else. Even in boom periods, our capitalist economy includes a lot of hidden unemployment. Eventually demand for workers grows strong enough to raise average wages, but recession arrives to raise unemployment and dampen wage growth. Recession flows from active government policy or overinvestment. In the '90s, those who ran the American economy seemed to fear inflation and higher wages more than recession.

Financial markets, complained economist Gordon Richards of the National Association of Manufacturers, "have a pathological fear of growth" (Rosenblatt, 1996; Silverstein, 2000). The Federal Reserve Board raised interest rates many times in 1994-1995 and in 1999-2000 to curb inflation and wage increases. Eventually the FRB reversed itself when autonomous factors sent the economy into a tailspin. An excess of shopping malls and dotcoms led to a falling stock market and rising unemployment. While the Fed tried to pump things up, the economy sank. September 11, 2001 was just the final blow. Whether by FRB action or the normal business cycle, recession arrives to recreate the labor surplus that keeps wages down and limits the creation of good regular jobs. Growth cannot permanently erase the job-related poverty and near poverty of the bottom fifth of our population because its success in raising wages incites the authorities to stop it.

Other rich capitalist economies have unemployment problems, but most have institutions and laws that compensate for the vulnerable position of employees in capitalist labor markets. Compensators include strong unions, extensive income supports, substantial unemployment insurance benefits, and political parties that support progressive taxation. In the U.S. in the 1980s and 1990s, unions weakened, Democrats became more subservient to big money, the minimum wage lagged, unemployment insurance coverage shrank, and tax policy often accentuated income inequality.

Tax policy, about which not much more will be said in this paper, is an outstanding example of the failure of anti-poverty politics and institutions to mitigate the inequalities that arise in our economy. Because of high unemployment, weaker unions, and a low minimum wage, average wages did not take off until the late 1990s (Figure 2). Meanwhile, because of the winner-take-all nature of American markets and because of corruption in the boardrooms, CEO pay jumped from 85 times to 326 times average pay between 1990 and 1997 (Anderson et al., 1999, p. 3). Without countervailing political action, almost all the gains of economic growth were skimmed off at the top. The amounts were huge. It used to be argued that if we redistributed the incomes of the rich, the poor would not get much because there were so many of them and so few rich Americans. But it is clear now that a lot of poverty could be solved by reversing our extremely unequal distribution of income. If we had redistributed just 42.5% of *one year's (1997 to 1998) increase* in the net worth of the 400 richest Americans, that $48.4 billion would have lifted thirty million Americans above the poverty line. As it was, nine-tenths of growth in the economic pie over 1977-1999 went to the top 1% of the households (Collins, Leondar-Wright, and Sklar, 1999, p. 17; Greenhouse, 2000, p. 3).

FIGURE 2. Real Average Hourly Earnings of American Workers, 1961-2001 (Production and Nonsupervisory Private Nonagricultural Employees)

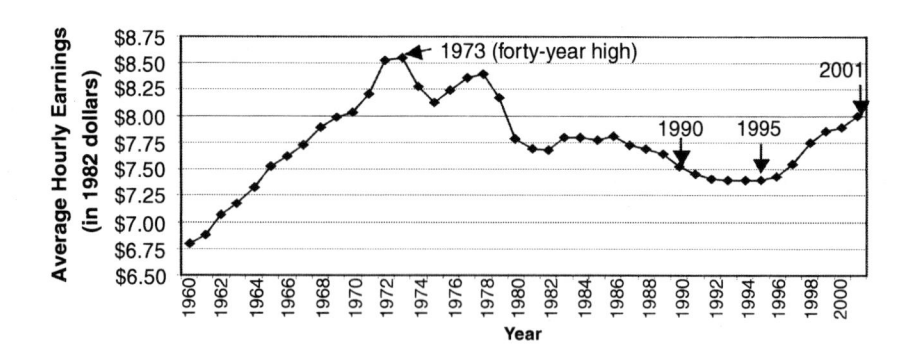

Source: *Economic report of the president* (2002) at http://w3.access.gpo.gov/usbudget/fy2003/sheets/b47.xls

The body of this paper sets out the details of the argument that welfare reform has been a failure and that economic growth cannot wipe out American poverty. The main argument is simple. The U.S. has a hugely flexible labor force and a mountain of hidden unemployment. These account for a good portion of the poverty and near poverty of those able to work. Substantial unemployment is the norm; recessions with higher unemployment are inevitable. Private markets cannot erase poverty.

SKILLS, POWER, AND INEQUALITY

Against my interpretation, there is an alternative, popular not only among conservatives, but also liberals and centrists like Bill Clinton, his first Secretary of Labor, Robert Reich, and many Americans. That is the argument that people have low incomes because they lack training and skills. We know that Michael Jordan was very talented and very well paid. We know that people with more schooling earn more than those with less. And we hear too that those who are trained for our high tech age will make out the best (Blank, 1997, pp. 65-68; Madrick, 1998a; Howell, 1994 and 2000).

Nevertheless, despite what these stories seem to tell us, the skills argument explains very little about why so many Americans are poor and nearly poor. Even Federal Reserve Chair Alan Greenspan admitted that we should look deeper than skill-biased technological explanations to fully understand growing wage inequalities (Bluestone and Harrison, 2001, p. 193). There are so many holes in the skills-and-education argument that, while it may tell us about Michael Jordan and nuclear physicists, it explains little about poverty. Consider these propositions:

1. While it is true that many jobs in America require specialized training, many require mainly what can be learned on the job. Economist Kenneth Arrow pointed out many years ago that much learning does not precede going to work "but is accomplished in the course of work" (Bluestone and Harrison, 2001, p. 77).
2. The '90s showed that when the economy grows fast enough, there are plenty of jobs for the less skilled. Economist Jeff Madrick (1998b, p. 60), noting the rise in wages for low-income workers in 1997-1998, argued that "so-called unskilled workers can handle their new jobs." But there has to be enough labor demand to force employers to start raising wages and increase hiring.
3. There are plenty of reasons to improve our schools–empowerment, citizenship, richer lives–but lifting people's educational and skill levels won't necessarily increase the number of high-skill jobs in the economy. In the '70s and '90s there was a glut of educated labor; the wages of new college graduates fell 7% over 1989-1997. Despite some gains in the '90s, in 1997 new engineers and scientists were earning 11% and 8% less than their counterparts in 1989. Frederick Pryor and David Schaffer (2000) showed that a recent excess of educated workers fell down into less skilled jobs, driving out less-skilled workers who were perfectly fit for those jobs. Others have pointed out that the big winners in the '90s were not scientists and high tech workers but doctors, lawyers, sales representatives, brokers and managers (Mishel et al., 1999, pp. 120-121; Tonelson, 2000, pp. 28ff. and 98ff.; Bluestone and Harrison, 2001, p. 193; Berg, 1971).
4. Many concrete examples suggest that the link between pay on the one hand and, on the other, skill level, efficiency, and social contribution is tenuous. It seems an axiom of free marketeers and human capital economists that people are paid what they are worth. But the reality is that many political, social, and economic factors shape compensation. We know, for example, that women and minorities are often paid less than others for the same contribution. We know that a substantial element in the determination of executive pay has

to do not with managerial skills but with the cozy relationship between boards of directors and managers; it is easy to cite examples of CEOs who failed miserably but walked away with huge bonuses and severance packages (Lublin, 1998, pp. R1-R14; Frank and Cook, 1996). As a third example, the share of child-care workers with more than a high school degree jumped from 18% to 42% (1984-1997), but real wages declined; more training yielded less pay (Howell, 2000, p. 77). Finally, stepping beyond the skill issue narrowly conceived, it is not a law of nature that those who know how to sweep the halls or take care of our children–and do a good job at it–must be paid poorly for their hard and often skillful work.

The widespread problem of low pay in the U.S. will not be fixed mainly by raising the average level of education and training; a higher average level of schooling may only intensify the game of musical chairs for too few good jobs. We need better incomes for some of the poor who cannot work for pay, but for millions of poor adults, we need, to paraphrase a Spike Lee movie, More Better Jobs.

COMPENSATORS AND TARGETED POLICIES: CLINTON'S FAIR RECORD

Before we examine welfare reform and labor markets, we discuss whether President Clinton supported specific measures to assist the poor. After the political disaster of health reform in 1993, Clinton's strategy was to take small steps. He supported the Children's Health Insurance Program cobbled together by Ted Kennedy and Orrin Hatch in 1997 to expand health care for poor children (Starr, 2000, pp. 18-19). He supported an increase in the federal minimum wage to $5.15 (1997). This helped the working poor a bit, but the new minimum was still 30% below its real level of the late 1960s, and it was not enough to lift any but small families over the poverty line. Local "living wage" ordinances that set pay rates at $7 to $10 an hour were more likely to do that, but no one in the Clinton administration got out in front of the living wage campaigns (Moberg, 2000).

Clinton's first effort on taxes was progressive. In 1993, rates were raised for the top fifth and especially the top one percent (some was given back in the Taxpayer Relief Act of 1997). Also Clinton supported an expansion of the Earned Income Tax Credit (EITC) which increased the number of covered families from 14 to 20 million (Pollin, 2000, p. 25).

EITC is a negative income tax. Improvements meant that a very low-income breadwinner with two or more dependents, forced off welfare by welfare reform, could combine minimum wage earnings ($10,000 for a person who worked full-time most of the year) with up to $3,656 in federal payments. She would fall thousands of dollars short of supplying her family's real needs but she might rise above the poverty line for a family of three ($13,133 in 1998). The president's economists claimed that EITC lifted 4.3 million Americans out of poverty in 1997, about twice as many as in 1993 (*Economic Report of the President*, 1999, pp. 112-114; Jencks, 1997, pp. 33-40). Finally, Clinton deflected conservative calls for privatizing Social Security; thereby he saved millions from falling into poverty later in this century, for Social Security lifts the elderly from being the poorest to one of the least poor social groups (Twentieth Century Fund, 1998, pp. 11-12).

Overall, Clinton made only a fair record. It was better than what had gone before when President Bush seemed indifferent to people's economic problems, but it was not an excellent record for a president who was elected because voters were anxious about low wages and high health care costs. Health care reform had been a campaign issue; its failure in 1993 meant continued insecurity for some forty million Americans, many of them the working poor who lacked any health insurance, private or public. Also, Clinton did nothing to reverse one of America's most important poverty policies of the 1980s and '90s: locking up young people from low-income backgrounds. Finally, although he won many union votes, Clinton did little to assist unionization; he offered little more than rhetoric to defend labor standards as he pushed for unregulated global capitalism. Overall, one economist concluded that Clinton had done "virtually nothing to advance the interests of organized labor or working people more generally" (Pollin, 2000, p. 20; Bluestone and Harrison, 2001, p. 15).

While Clinton seemed more compassionate toward the poor than Ronald Reagan, the different effects on poor people of each man's two-term presidency were not as large as one might expect. Reagan cut welfare spending a bit; Clinton encouraged the forces that eliminated the federal welfare entitlement. The statistical record of the Clinton years was not so much better than Reagan's: poverty rates averaged 13.2% during Clinton's terms (1993-2000) and 14.1% during Reagan's (1981-1988). It is true that poverty rates reached a thirty-year low in 1999-2000 (U.S. Bureau of the Census, 2001). And Clinton must look good to poor people now, against the second George Bush, who offers only the rhetoric of compassion and more tax cuts for the affluent. But Clinton probably left office just in time, just before his luck ran out; his neo-liberal approach to poverty had just about run its course and some kind of recession with more poverty was in store, regardless of who was in office.

WELFARE REPEAL: IGNORING LABOR MARKETS

Whatever sound reasons there were for welfare reform, they were not the main ones in play when Aid to Families with Dependent Children (AFDC) was repealed in August of 1996. Conservatives had been trying for years to get rid of AFDC. The 1996 law showed that conservative ideas had won, for it reflected the views of Ronald Reagan and Charles Murray that poverty was not a matter of low wages and unemployment, of structured economic inequalities (around class, race, and gender), and a miserly welfare state. Rather, it stemmed from welfare dependence and liberal permissiveness. By the mid-90s most Republicans and many Democrats had jumped on this bandwagon. It did not matter that the average size of welfare families was shrinking or that millions went on and off the rolls as the job market rose and fell. The idea of a permanent population of lazy welfare recipients won out. Newt Gingrich led the charge but Clinton signed the Personal Responsibility and Work Opportunity Reconciliation Act (Bryner, 1998, pp. 11, 17, 67-78, 107, 152; Reagan, 1986; Pierson, 1995, pp. 115-128; Gillespie and Schellhas, 1994, pp. 65-77, 169-196).

The politics of the Personal Responsibility and Work Opportunity Reconciliation Act (PRWORA) ignored facts and dehumanized welfare recipients. During Congressional debate, Florida's John Mica compared welfare recipients to wild animals and held up a sign that read: "Don't Feed the Alligators" (Bryner, 1998, pp. 114-115). Champions of welfare reform suppressed the fact that millions of working Americans were poor. Centrists and liberals who agreed to welfare reform hoping to get big job and training programs did not get very much (Edleman, 1997; Piven & Ellwood, 1996).

Under the new law, no family could get federal funds for welfare beyond five years. States could limit welfare to fewer than five years. States were encouraged to force recipients off welfare into the work force, regardless of training or mental health or child-care issues. The law made it very difficult for immigrants to get welfare, food stamps, and disability payments. It cut support for disabled children. There were no provisions for funding increases during recessions (Public Law 104-193, 1996; Bryner, pp. 185-182; Cammisa, 1998, pp. 117-131; Kilbourn, 2001).

The focus of PRWORA was to get poor people off the public purse; the alleviation of poverty was not even an express purpose of the law. While it is too soon in 2002 to make a final judgement on welfare reform, it is clear that if the goal was to cut people from the rolls, reform succeeded. The numbers fell by half and in Wisconsin by 90%. Some former welfare mothers at work felt better about themselves because they were self-supporting. Others did not. In one survey of leavers, 69% said life was better, but 69% said they were barely making ends meet (Brauner and Loprest, 1999, p. 8).

At least in the short run, and even before the recession of 2001-2002 wrecked the job market, welfare reform was failing in three significant ways. First, in most states not much had been done to repair the problems that limited poor people's success in the world. People were pushed into jobs, any jobs; training and general education were downplayed. By the middle of 1999, Los Angeles County had only 150 people in its federally funded training program; thousands were eligible. Second, to the extent that poor people were trapped in bad family and neighborhood situations—mental illness, drug addiction, alcoholism, abusive relationships, serious physical and psychological disabilities—welfare reform failed. These kinds of problems were typical of the long-term welfare recipients who were allegedly the target of welfare reform; but PRWORA and the states did little to address them. Almost nothing was done for fathers in poverty (Foster, 2000; Goldstein, 2000; "States Lag," 1999; Bane, 1997; Blank, 1997, pp. 42-47; Rivera, 2001; Simon, 2001). And third, most welfare clients who took jobs were as poor as they had been on welfare. They lost welfare payments, rent supplements and, eventually, Medicaid; and they faced new transportation, childcare, and clothing costs (DeParle, 1999; Albelda, 1999; Mistrano, 1999; Houppert, 1999).

A final analysis of the effects of welfare repeal would have to follow welfare leavers carefully and systematically over many years, through economic expansion and recession. We know that the recession of 2001-2002 had a devastating impact on ex-welfare clients and low-income workers in general (Peterson, 2001). But even earlier reports, during a strong job market, were not encouraging. One national sample of those who left over 1995-1997 showed that a fifth were without work, a working spouse, or government disability support, almost a third had returned to welfare, and the rest were working at low-wage jobs that paid $6.61 an hour and $1,149 a month. On the plus side, half the leavers still had Medicaid (Loprest, 1999). An Illinois survey of those leaving welfare from mid-1997 though December of 1998 found 64% living in poverty (Armato, 2000). Welfare reform in Wisconsin won Tommy Thompson the position as George W. Bush's Secretary of Health and Human Services, but in the first three years of "Wisconsin Works," one-fourth of ex-welfare recipients were back on the rolls and half of those at work were in poverty. As recession arrived, unemployment rose to 7.6% in Milwaukee; Wisconsin's welfare rolls jumped by 25% in less than a year. One scholarly report claimed that there were seven job seekers for every job in Milwaukee's core. Yet Wisconsin's welfare reformers stayed hard-hearted: cash aid would only make the poor lazy–even those who had recently been working (Associated Press, 2001; Simon, 2001).

Leaving welfare meant more poverty for some of the poorest Americans. The average incomes of the poorest 20% of all American female-headed families with children fell $580 between 1995 and 1997, largely due to cuts in government cash and food assistance. For the 20% of female-headed families right at the poverty line, earnings increased substantially but the loss of benefits left them as poor as before (Center on Budget and Policy Priorities, 1999; Jencks and Swingle, 2000). In September of 2001, Secretary Thompson boasted that welfare reform had "helped unprecedented numbers of people on welfare to become self-supporting," but that was a cruel half-truth. Many who had been poor on welfare were now poor off welfare. Over 1995-2000 the poorest 40% of single mothers increased their annual earnings by $2,300, but their disposable income increased by only $292 because they lost welfare benefits and food stamps (Jackson, 2001; Harden, 2001).

In South Carolina, which every month offered welfare recipients $201 in cash and $329 in food stamps ($6,300 a year), perhaps it was possible to be better off without welfare. But in many places the situation of ex-recipients deteriorated. In Milwaukee, homeless shelters ran out of room in the winter of 1998-1999. A year later in San Diego more of the homeless were single-parent families and there was not enough space for them in local shelters. This occurred in the midst of the longest economic expansion in American history. Boosters of ending welfare ignored the fact that work could not cure poverty for many people. In 1998, the number of Americans working full-time, year-round, but still poor, rose by 20% or by 459,000 people. This was not a large fraction of the American population but that it was rising in a boom time was shocking (Edelhoch, 1999; Collins and Goldberg, 1999; Piven, 1999; Massing, 1999; Perry, 2000; Pollin, 2000, p. 26).

Some welfare reforms looked effective and evaluators strained to give them a positive spin. One favorably reviewed program was the Minnesota Family Investment Program (MFIP); its creators intended that it would solve poverty as well as get people off welfare. MFIP encouraged work by allowing recipients to keep more of their benefits after they started working until their income reached 140% of the poverty line. The results were positive, but not as stunning as the evaluators claimed. More people in the MFIP group worked after three years than in the regular AFDC group (50% vs. 37%); but earnings in both groups were still extremely low (on an annualized basis $3,820 and $3,116). Although MFIP got more work out of some recipients, some adults in two-parent families worked less to devote more time to family. By and large, the gains were significant in percentage terms but the dollar amounts were miserable. MFIP had not solved much poverty (Berlin, 2000; Cimons, 2000; Knox, Miller, and Gennetian, 2000).

But for many politicians and propagandists, welfare repeal was not about solving poverty; it aimed to get people off the public rolls and under market discipline (Murray, 1984). And it was very effective in that respect. This central objective of welfare reform was successful, in part because there was a booming economy in which jobs appeared to be plentiful, and in part because conservative ideas ruled the day. These two things made it easier to push people off welfare and keep people off welfare. If welfare clients were politically isolated–and they were, in part because of the triumph of conservative ideas about welfare, but also because the idea of paying mothers to stay home looked unfair when many non-poor mothers were at work–it was easy to fix welfare: kick people off welfare and keep them off. Federal law set an upward limit of five years; but some states imposed shorter time limits and some agencies made it very difficult for poor people to get on welfare. New York City and Mississippi and Idaho led the way. South Carolina officials ejected families from welfare for a single act of noncompliance, such as being late for an appointment (Houppert, 1999; Green, 2000, pp. 33, 38).

So millions of people who would once have been poor on welfare were poor off welfare. Nothing structural had been done to fix the low-wage problem and despite all the hype about a high tech society, the economy continued to generate huge numbers of low-wage jobs (Greenhouse, 2000). Even strong supporters of government income programs knew that the American welfare system was degrading, demoralizing, financially inadequate, and politically divisive and needed repair. But there were few liberal voices arguing that Americans should *enrich* income-support systems *and fix* the poverty-wage labor market. Many Democrats, like their leader in the White House, seemed to accept the conservative analysis that blamed welfare for poverty and family breakups. But welfare reform made things worse by tossing two million workers into the low-wage pool. This helped to keep wage levels low. Despite occasional rhetoric from both parties in the late '90s about a second hike in the minimum wage, nothing happened. Less energy was expended on solving poverty than on ending welfare.

THE HIDDEN LABOR FORCE, OR WHY POVERTY WON'T GO AWAY

Economic growth has been America's preferred method of solving poverty; it is politically easier than taking from the rich and giving to the poor. A rising tide is said to lift all boats. And it worked in the 1950s and 1960s, when an unusual mix of government policy, world conditions, and spending surges from two wars slashed poverty rates. In the 1990s, however, growth was not having the same effect. Early in the decade there was talk of the jobless recovery, and poverty rates did not fall until 1994 and then only slowly (Figure 1). Poverty expert Rebecca Blank and others argued that in the new economy there was less demand for unskilled workers, but neither she nor others proved the case (Miller, 1994; Tonelson, 2000, pp. 19-23). I believe the problem was bigger. It is true that those with fewer "skills" and educational credentials earned less, but the more fundamental problem was a work force traumatized by decades of layoffs and insecurity, a persistent labor surplus, and continuing weakness in institutions like unions and income-support programs that compensate for the harsh economics of the labor market. Much of what follows in this section suggests that wages did not rise and poverty did not fall as fast as we would have predicted in a high-growth, full-employment economy because there was a great deal of hidden unemployment.

Analyzing the links among poverty, work, and economic growth is a way to judge both the record of the Clinton years and the viability of the growth cure for poverty. As a campaigner, Clinton had promised public investment, infrastructure repair, support for skill improvement, and job creation. In *Putting People First*, he proposed spending $50 billion a year for four years in these areas. But Alan Greenspan, deficit hawks in Congress, and Wall Street advisors convinced the president to set aside his economic stimulus plan. He had hoped, he told the American people on February 15, 1993, "to invest in your future by creating jobs, expanding education, reforming health care. . . . But I can't–because the deficit has increased so much beyond my earlier estimates. . . ." So the administration pulled out all the stops to pass, without Republican votes, a plan to reduce the deficit by raising taxes and cutting spending. In effect, Clinton cleaned up Reagan's mess and pampered Wall Street and Greenspan in hopes that low interest rates would nurture strong economic growth. Later, when Clinton tried to get Congressional approval for a modest stimulus package, Republicans filibustered it to death (Jones, 1996, p. 29; Reich, 1997, pp. 26-31; Bluestone and Harrison, 2001, pp. 13-15, 118ff).

Perhaps Wall Street and Skid Row had common interests. Were low-income Americans the beneficiaries of solid growth? As it turned out, economic growth rates were good, although sluggish at first. In the first six years of Clinton's presidency, real Gross Domestic Product, a common measure of total output, grew a total 25%, not as good as JFK-LBJ's first six years (36%) but better than equivalent periods under Reagan (22%) and Eisenhower (17.5%) (U.S. Department of Commerce, Bureau of Economic Analysis). For the first time in many years, unemployment rates approached 4%, which many economists considered a sign of full employment.

Yet strong economic growth was slow to bring equivalent gains against poverty and low wages (Figures 1 and 2). Not until four or five years after expansion began in 1991 did wages really start climbing. The share of all jobs paying poverty-level wages still stood at 26.8% in 1999; it had been 28.5% in 1989 and 23.7% in 1979 (Mishel, Bernstein, and Schmitt, 2001, p. 130). The slow pace of lifting low-wage workers indicated that something was going on below the surface, something that full-employment statistics missed.

Wages did begin responding to the boom in the second half of the '90s, but when growth stopped in 2001, average pay still had not caught up with previous highs. That was not only because, as we shall see, there were few real labor shortages but also because when they needed workers, employers tried everything to avoid wage increases. They offered new employees free transportation, tuition subsidies, shopping discounts, and softball fields before they increased pay. Frank L. Salizzoni, chief executive at H&R Block, claimed, "We have not been pressured to raise wages because of the labor shortage." Even when employers had to increase pay to attract workers, they did not go far. When Sprint lost operators to better jobs, the company had to increase hourly pay from $7 to $8.25 to get replacements, but the latter rate was still just around the federal poverty line for a family of four (Uchitelle, 2000; Gosselin, 1999b, Hirsch, 2000).

Given the slow reaction of wages, it would have taken a very long boom to lift the bottom, and the lifting had just begun when the Federal Reserve Board began raising interest rates in the summer of 1999 to slow the economy. And since certain groups started far back, it would have taken a much longer and deeper boom than even the record Clinton expansion to solve their poverty. Jobs had grown by 7.5% for blacks and 14% for Latinos, faster than for whites. By the late '90s, reported unemployment rates for these groups were at their lowest level since the data were first collected in 1972. But they still remained higher at 8.1% and 5.8% than the rates for whites. Recession increased minority jobless rates rapidly; by November of 2001 black rates were 10.1% and Latino rates 7.6% (the U.S. rate was 5.7%) (Gosselin, 1999a; Vieth, 2001). And these rates understated unemployment.

The problem was not limited to minorities. Most workers, white and black, had seen a long-term wage decline from the mid-70s to the mid-90s. Some did worse than others. Female workers still earned less than males, but they were gaining; they lost less in the early '90s and gained more in the late '90s. The median real hourly wage of male workers fell 9.1% over 1979-1989, fell again by 6.5% over 1989-1995, and then increased by 5.5% over 1995-1999. The last was good news, but still less than half the previous losses. High school graduates with no college experience (males and females) experienced a real wage decline over 1979-1995 of 15%; things turned around for them but not by much: their wage rates rose a total of 4.4% over 1995-1999 (Mishel et al., 2001, pp. 125-127, 157; *Economic Report of the President*, 1999). In terms of median annual earnings of full-time, full-year workers, by 1997, women's pay had grown only by 3% over 1989 levels, and men's was still 4% below the 1989 level (Economic Policy Institute, 1999; Osterman, 1999, p. 74).

What was wrong? The labor market of 1993-2000 seemed ideal: strong growth and low inflation. For orthodox economists, the happy mystery was not why so many stayed poor but why low unemployment had not led to generalized labor shortages and surging wages. The press did report spot shortages in some occupations and some states, but "We seem to keep finding the bodies to hire," as UC Berkeley economist Bradford DeLong put it (Gosselin, 1999a, p. A30; Lee, 1998a; Lee, 1999; Silverstein, 1998). That was a surprise. Officially, the civilian labor force increased by about 10%, well below increases of 16% in the 1960s and 1980s and 27% in the 1970s. In part slow growth in the official labor force reflected demographic factors, for the adult population had not grown very fast (8.5%) compared, for example, to the 1970s (18%). But demand for labor grew slowly also. For much of the decade, adult labor force participation rates, while high, did not grow much either, rising from 66.5% to 67.1% (1990-1998), a slight decline for men almost offsetting a small increase for women. Apparently, until late in the decade, demand for labor was not very strong. Once demand picked up, there were plenty of workers (*Economic Report of the President*, 1999, pp. 368-377).

Wages did not grow very fast and economic growth cured less poverty than it once had for three pivotal reasons. First, deregulation, weakening unions, and inadequate income programs like unemployment insurance meant that employees operated in a more harshly competitive market than they had in the 1950s and '60s. Second, workers were traumatized by recent history–greater job insecurity and weaker social programs–and government did little to counteract these facts. Just the opposite. Democrats and Republicans alike did more to subject workers to a global "free market." Third, there were usually enough workers for most of the jobs offered. Widely publicized unemployment rates underestimated the available labor supply and supported fears about labor shortages which, in the late '90s, incited the Federal Reserve Board to raise interest rates and expand the labor surplus. Higher unemployment normally keeps wages down. The rest of this section focuses on the second and third of these factors. As to the second, workers' sense of insecurity reflected reality. While official unemployment rates were low, layoffs continued at a high rate (Lee, 1998b). In the '70s, 67% of all workers stayed with one employer at least nine years; in the '80s, 52%. The percentage of workers who lost their jobs in the early years of the Clinton recovery (1993-1995) was 11.4%, almost as bad as the 12.3% level reached in the 1981-1983 depression (Mishel et al., 1999, p. 235). Even the president's economists admitted in 1999 that "job displacement remains relatively high given today's low unemployment rates" (*Economic Report of the President*, 1999, p. 126). Layoffs were becoming the "Strategy of First Resort." A sampling of the press in 1998, a prosperous year, found almost forty announcements that giant corporations like Exxon, Packard Bell, Boeing, and Raytheon were each laying off thousands of workers. Adding to job anxieties was the fact that only a third of the unemployed were receiving unemployment insurance (Osterman, 1999, pp. 49-53, 125; Pollin, 2000, p. 39; Maharaj, 1998; Jacoby, 1998).

Also making employees nervous was growth in the contingent labor force. Those counted as temporary workers had expanded by a factor of ten since 1973; by the turn of the century, they comprised 2 1/2% of the labor force. This seemed a tiny fraction, but as economist Paul Osterman noted, "regular employees are well aware of contingent employment within their organization and the implicit threat it entails" (Osterman, 1999, pp. 45-58; Mishel et al., 1999, pp. 226-250). Other threats were common too. Labor expert Kate Bronfenbrenner found that more than half the firms she surveyed fought unionization by threatening to shut down U.S. operations (Tonelson, 2000, p. 47).

These things made American workers less aggressive and glad to have a job. But the main force that dampened employee bargaining power–what made people's feelings of insecurity very real–was the fact that the potential labor force was much larger than official data showed and unemployment was much higher than the official unemployment rate. While the federal government's most highly publicized model of the labor force includes only those who are at work and those who are actively looking for work, there also is a very large group of workers in what I call the Nearby Labor Force (NLF). It is because this Nearby Labor Force was outside the official one that unemployment looked low, and it is because its members were ready to take jobs as conditions and pay improved that wages did not rise very much for very long.[1]

It is not possible to quantify precisely the real American labor force and real unemployment in the 1990s. But we can outline groups that are not included in the officially unemployed, people who are employed but seeking more work, and workers that seem distant from the American labor force but have an impact on employee bargaining power. Together, they comprise a very large group.

1. First, the officially unemployed. These are people who have searched for work in the weeks preceding the monthly unemployment survey. They were about 6% of the labor force in the mid-90s and 4% by the late '90s. Using only this group, the unemployment problem appeared to be over by the late '90s. But to these people, who accounted for widely publicized monthly national unemployment rates, I would add many other categories.
2. Millions of part-time workers who want full-time work can be considered partially unemployed. There were almost five million of them in 1995 (Bluestone and Harrison, 2001, p. 98).
3. At different points in the business cycle hundreds of thousands and sometimes more than a million Americans are "discouraged" workers who want to work but have given up looking and are not counted as unemployed. When the categories of involuntary part-timers and discouraged workers are included, the national unemployment rate is often double the official rate, about 10% in 2000.[2]
4. To these categories–and involving some duplication with previous categories–we must add people who were always about to be available for work because the rapid pace of "downsizing" was

eliminating their jobs. In 1993-1994, 6.5 million employees had their jobs wiped out and although most found work again, by 1996 1.5 million had not and .5 million were only working part-time. Some of these downsized workers must have stopped looking for work and were not counted as unemployed (Osterman, 1999, p. 285).
5. Many of the urban poor were outside the labor force and not counted as unemployed. Some were being counted in the late '90s as unemployment declined (Uchitelle, 2000).
6. The number of immigrants flowing into the labor force continued to be very high in the '90s (Lee, 1999; Tonelson, 2000, p. 48).
7. Several million women were thrown off welfare and into the work force as a result of the 1996 repeal of Aid to Families with Dependent Children.
8. More older Americans wanted to return to work. A Harris poll found that four million older Americans wanted jobs. There were 18 million Americans ages 65-74 who were not in hospitals or nursing homes; only 3 million had jobs ("Employment's New Age," 2000; Bluestone and Harrison, 2001, p. 246).
9. The male segment of the prison population equaled 2.3% of the potential male labor force. Had they been out of prison, many would have shown up as unemployed. Some were in prison because of dim employment prospects (Western, 2001, pp. 31-36).
10. There were uncounted numbers of scientists and engineers whom labor-short companies rejected because they required company training to adapt their skills to new jobs; instead of paying for training or improving pay to attract workers, employers used a special immigration program (H-1B) to import cheaper workers. H-1B immigration continued even as the high tech sector sank and layoffs soared (Girion, 2000; Shriver, 2001).
11. Existing employees, to compensate for slow wage growth or fearful of losing their jobs, raised their hours of work in the '90s by an amount equivalent to an increase in the labor force of 3% or 4% (Bluestone and Rose, 1998).
12. Many temporary workers were not counted as unemployed when they were between jobs; and millions of independent contractors, often downsized professionals, were unemployed but too proud to admit it (Bluestone and Harrison 2001, p. 98; Thurow, 1996, p. 56).
13. Finally, the American labor force was increasingly integrated into the worldwide labor force, not only by immigration, but by the

ease with which American companies sent work abroad. Nations with huge populations and staggering unemployment rates like India and China functioned as an adjunct to the American labor force. Business writers William Wolman and Anne Colamosca claimed that each American competed with 2.8 inhabitants of the industrialized world in 1989; in 1994 each competed with 21 people around the world (Tonelson, 2000, pp. 53-80).

The sheer number of additional categories of ready workers suggests a giant, accordion-like labor force, expanding now at the top, now at the bottom as the music of demand directed. Other experts have arrived at similarly high estimates for real unemployment. In the mid-90s, Lester Thurow (1996) found an "enormous sea of unemployment and underemployment," with a third of the American work force looking for jobs or more hours. Marc-Andre Pigeon and L. Randall Wray (1999) argued that the Clinton boom had not tightened labor markets enough to draw in many of those with lower schooling. If labor markets had really been tight, more of those without college education would have been pulled up the job ladder. In light of estimates like Thurow's, Pigeon and Wray's, and my own, it is realistic to think that unemployment was closer to 10% or 20% than 5%. And if real unemployment were so large, we know why, at the end of the longest economic expansion in American history, a tenth of the population was still poor even by government standards, another tenth was near poor, and American wages had not recovered much that had been lost since the early 1970s.

I have told the unemployment story for the good times of the '90s. But even as good times got better and wages finally increased several years in a row, the monetary authorities raised interest rates six times in 1999-2000 to halt job growth. For fear of inflation and of wages that ate into profits, a government agency strived to halt the economic expansion which, according to many conservatives and some liberals, was the best way to solve poverty through work. Rising average wages, which had begun to cure poverty, were precisely the signal that growth had to be curbed.

CONCLUSION

Recessions, which generate unemployment and poverty, have various causes. The Federal Reserve Board tried to create one in 1999-2000 and then, when autonomous forces in the economy deteriorated, it backtracked. But the seeds of recession sprouted in 2001 and the terrorist attacks of September 2001 made things worse. The result was more unemployment, an end to wage gains for most workers, and, it seems certain, more poverty.

The main point to keep in mind is that conservatives and centrists have promised something they refuse to deliver. They claim that employment is the main salvation of the poor–hence the repeal of AFDC and the stingy American system of unemployment insurance–but they ask us to accept that the reasons this growth strategy has not worked for thirty years are the fault of the poor or an accident of history. But, in fact, it appears that American leaders will never allow the economy to run hot enough to cure unemployment and lift enough low-wage workers to wipe out job-related poverty.

One point of this paper is to argue for the creation of more and better jobs. Since most businesses are committed to a policy of worker insecurity, to job and wage cuts rather than job enrichment, enough good jobs for low- and middle-income Americans must come from government. But even if millions of jobs are some day created by public agencies, the working poor need immediate improvements in the minimum wage and the Earned Income Tax Credit, substantial subsidies for health insurance and child care, and a renaissance in the living wage and union movements.

On a more profound level, Americans need to debate poverty, leisure, and affluence. Our goal should not be to create an economy in which every single employable person is working full-time. That is impossible and undesirable. Income must be more fairly distributed. Those at the bottom and middle need higher pay and families need to be able to decide that only one family member will work or that both will work less. We need to debate our lack of public support for caregivers. This debate would synthesize concerns of the 1950s and '60s with concerns of the 1980s and '90s.

American capitalism does not produce more poverty than most rich nations, but the U.S. does less to help its poor than fourteen other rich nations (Figure 3). Prior to government programs (lefthand column), the U.S. does not have the highest poverty rate, but once the impact of government programs is included, it does. Until unions and similar organizations are more powerful and until the American welfare state is fixed, the U.S. will continue to have among the highest poverty rates of all the rich nations. The explanation for high poverty rates in America is not to be found in the details of this or that program or in the bad attitudes of poor people, but in a labor market dominated by employers and a political process that allows a severe maldistribution of income. Other rich capitalist

FIGURE 3. Relative Poverty Rates Before and After Government Programs, 1991

	Pre-tax & pre-transfer payments poverty rates	Post-tax & post-transfer payments poverty rates
Australia	21.3%	6.4%
Belgium	23.9%	2.2%
Canada	21.6%	5.6%
Denmark	23.9%	3.5%
Finland	9.8%	2.3%
France	27.5%	4.8%
Germany	14.1%	2.4%
Ireland	25.8%	4.7%
Italy	21.8%	5.0%
Netherlands	20.5%	4.3%
Norway	9.3%	1.7%
Sweden	20.6%	3.8%
Switzerland	12.8%	4.3%
United Kingdom	25.7%	5.3%
United States	21.0%	11.7%

Source: Adapted from Table 3, Kenworthy (1998), by permission of author.

nations have similar problems, but somewhere in their past, they had political and union movements that built compensators against the inegalitarian effects of the market system. The U.S. has more poverty and its low-income citizens are more insecure because the U.S. is organizationally and politically backward. It is an old story but still true.

NOTES

1. For economists, the late '90s raised a question about NAIRU, the Non-Accelerating Inflation Rate of Unemployment. Especially conservatives had argued that once unemployment dipped below 6% or 7%, wages and inflation would take off; this was used as an argument against robust economic growth. But in the '90s unemployment fell far below 6% without much inflation. From one angle, NAIRU appeared to be dead, but if I am right, the Nearby Labor Force saves some of NAIRU.

2. The Labor Department and Census Bureau have developed more expansive unemployment figures. U-6, which includes discouraged workers and part-timers wanting full-time work, doubles the unemployment rate. These higher rates are not widely publicized. An exception is Uchitelle (2000), who noted that in February of

2000, there were 6 million unemployed workers looking for work, 4 million who wanted to work but were not looking, 3 million who had part-time work and wanted full-time work, and millions more who would enter the labor force under the right conditions.

REFERENCES

Albelda, R. (1999, January-February). What welfare reform has wrought. *Dollars and Sense*, 15-17.

Anderson, S., Cavanagh, J., Estes, R., Institute for Policy Studies, Collins, C., Hartman, C., & United for a Fair Economy (1999). *A decade of executive excess: The 1990s*. Boston, MA: United for a Fair Economy.

Armato, S. (2000, January). *Executive summary of "Living with welfare reform: A survey of low-income families in Illinois."* at http://www.workwelfareandfamilies.org/execsum.html.

Associated Press (2001, April 12). Wisconsin welfare reform a mixed bag, study shows. *Los Angeles Times*, p. A31.

Auletta, K. (1983). *The Underclass*. NY: Vintage Books.

Bane, M. J. (1997, January-February). Welfare as we might know it. *The American Prospect, 30*, 47-53.

Berg, I. (1971). *Education and jobs: The great training robbery*. Boston: Beacon Press.

Berlin, G. L. (2000, June 19-July 3). Welfare that works: Lessons from three experiments that fight dependency and poverty by rewarding work. *The American Prospect, 11*, 68-73.

Blank, R.M. (1997). *It takes a nation: A new agenda for fighting poverty*. Princeton: Princeton University Press.

Bluestone, B., & Harrison, B. (2001). *Growing prosperity: The battle for growth with equity in the 21st century*. Berkeley, CA: University of California Press.

Bluestone, B., & Rose, S. (1998). *The unmeasured labor force: The growth in work hours*. Annandale-on-Hudson, NY: Jerome Levy Economics Institute, Bard College.

Brauner, S., & Loprest, P. (1999, May). Where are they now? What states' studies of people who left welfare tell us. Assessing the New Federalism Project, No. A-32. DC: The Urban Institute.

Bryner, G. (1998). *Politics and public morality: The great American welfare reform debate*. NY: W.W. Norton and Co.

Cammisa, A. M. (1998). *From rhetoric to reform: Welfare policy in American politics*. Boulder, CO: Westview Press.

Center on Budget and Policy Priorities (1999). Average incomes of very poor families fell during early years of welfare reform, study finds, at www.cbpp.org./8-22-99wel.htm.

Cimons, M. (2000, June 1). Welfare plan gives families surer footing, study says. *Los Angeles Times*, pp. A1, A21;

Collins, C., Leondar-Wright, B., & Sklar, H. (1999). *Shifting fortunes: The perils of the growing American wealth gap*. Boston: United for a Fair Economy.

Collins, S., & Goldberg, G. S. (1999, Spring). South Carolina's welfare reform: More rough than right. *Social Policy, 29*, 16-33.

DeParle, J. (1999, December 30). Bold effort leaves much unchanged for the poor. *New York Times*, pp. A1, A12-A13.
Economic Policy Institute (1999). Jobless gaps still wide despite strong recovery. *Quarterly Wage and Employment Series, 3*, at epinet.org.
Economic report of the president (1999). Washington, DC: GPO.
Economic report of the president (2002), at http://w3access.gop.gov/usbudget/fy2003/shets/b47.xls.
Edelhoch, M. (1999, Spring). Welfare reform in South Carolina: "Roughly right." *Social Policy, 29*, 7-14.
Edelman, P. (1997, March). The worst thing Bill Clinton has done. *Atlantic Monthly*, 43-58.
Employment's new age (2000, July 30). *New York Times*, Sect. 4, p. 14.
Foster, H. (2000, May 26). Hard reality of welfare reform surfaces as caseloads creep up. *Seattle Post Intelligencer*, at http://seattlep-i.nwsource.com/local/welf26.shtml.
Frank, R. H., & Cook, P. J. (1996). *The Winner-Take-All Society*. NY: Penguin Books.
Galbraith, J. K. (1998). *Created unequal: The crisis in American pay*. NY: The Free Press.
Gillispie, E., & Shellhas, B. (Eds.). (1994). *Contract with America: The bold plan by Rep. Newt Gingrich, Rep. Dick Armey, and the House Republicans to change the nation*. NY: Random House.
Girion, L. (2000, September 4). Millions of jobless are uncounted, new study says. *Los Angeles Times*, pp. C1-C2.
Goldstein, A. (2000, June 1). Welfare reform's progress is stalled. *Washington Post*, at http://washingtonpost.com/wp-dyn/articles/A13355-2000May26.html.
Gosselin, P. G. (1999a, April 11). A rising tide puts the nation to work. *Los Angeles Times*, pp. A1, A30.
Gosselin, P. G. (1999b, August 30). Job picture still rosy as hiring gets creative. *Los Angeles Times*, pp. A1, A15.
Green, J. (2000, June 19-July 3). Holding out; Tough sanctions, tough luck. *The American Prospect, 11*, 33, 38.
Greenhouse, S. (2000, September 3). A rising tide, but some boats rise higher than others. *New York Times*, Week Section, p. 3.
Harden, B. (2001, August 12). 2-Parent families rise after change in welfare laws. *New York Times*, Section I, pp. 1, 24.
Houppert, K. (1999, October 25). You're not entitled! Welfare 'reform' is leading to government lawlessness. *The Nation*, 17.
Howell, D.R. (1994, Summer). The skills myth. *The American Prospect, 18*, 81-94.
Howell, D.R. (2000, June 19-July 3). Skills and the wage collapse. *The American Prospect, 11*, 74- 77.
Jackson, R.L. (2001, September 6). Family welfare rolls show slight drop. *Los Angeles Times*, p. A14.
Jacoby, S. M. (1998). Most workers find a sense of security in corporate life. *Los Angeles Times*, p. B5.
Jencks, C. (1997, May-June). The hidden paradox of welfare reform. *The American Prospect, 32*, 33- 40.

Jencks. C., & Swingle, J. (2000, January 3). Without a net: Whom the new welfare law helps and hurts. *The American Prospect, 11,* 37-41.

Jones, C.O. (1996). Campaigning to govern: The Clinton style. In C. Campbell and B. A. Rockman (Eds.), *The Clinton Presidency: First Appraisals* (pp. 15-50). Chatham, NJ: Chatham House.

Kenworthy, L. (1998). *Do social welfare policies reduce poverty? A cross-national assessment.* (Working Paper No. 188). Luxembourg Income Study.

Kilbourn, P.T. (2001, December 9). Recession is stretching the limit on welfare benefits. *New York Times,* p. A28.

Knox, V., Miller, C., & Gennetian, L. A. (2000). Reforming welfare and rewarding work: A summary of the final report on the Minnesota Family Investment Program, at http://www.mdrc.org/Reports2000/MFIP/MFIPSummary.htm.

Lee, D. (1998a, September 23). Labor supply falling short. *Los Angeles Times,* pp. D1, D6.

Lee, D. (1998b, November 11). 2 years, 6 layoffs, zero expectations. *Los Angeles Times,* pp. C1, C7.

Lee, D. (1999, December 7). Labor pinch has midwest pitching woo. *Los Angeles Times,* pp. A1, A24.

Loprest, P. (1999, August). How families that left welfare are doing: A national picture. Assessing the New Federalism Project, No. B1. DC: The Urban Institute.

Lubin, J. S. (1998, April 9). Pay for no performance. *Wall Street Journal,* pp. R1-R14.

Madrick, J. (1998a, March 26). Computers: Waiting for the revolution. *New York Review of Books,* 29-33.

Madrick, J. (1998b, November-December). The treadmill economy. *The American Prospect, 41,* 56- 60.

Maharaj, D. (1998, November 11). Layoffs: A company's strategy of first resort. *Los Angeles Times,* pp. C1, C7.

Mangum, G., Sum, A, & Fogg, N. (2000, March-April). Poverty ain't what it used to be. *Challenge: A Magazine of Economic Affairs, 43,* 97-103.

Massing, M. (1999, October 7). The end of welfare? *New York Review Books,* 22-27.

Miller, J. (1994, May-June). 1994, as the economy expands, opportunity contracts. *Dollars and Sense,* 8-11.

Mishel, L., Bernstein, J., & Schmitt, J. (1999). *The state of working America, 1998-1999.* Ithaca, NY: Cornell University Press.

Mishel, L., Bernstein, J., & Schmitt, J. (2001). *The state of working America, 2000/2001.* Ithaca, NY: Cornell University Press.

Mistrano, S. (1999, July 16). Welfare clock will run out before job supply catches up. *Los Angeles Times,* p. B7.

Moberg, D. (2000, June 19-July 3). Martha Jernegons's new shoes. *The American Prospect, 11,* 50-53.

Murray, C. (1984). *Losing ground: American social policy, 1950-1980.* NY: Basic Books.

Murray, C. (1999, November-December). And now for the bad news. *Commentary, 37,* 12-15.

Newton, J. (2000, December 8). Program to help poor buy homes is unveiled. *Los Angeles Times,* pp. B1, B7.

Osterman, P. (1999). *Securing prosperity: The American labor market: How it has changed and what to do about it.* Princeton, NJ: Princeton University Press.
Perry, T. (2000, January 24). Rise in homeless families strains San Diego aid. *Los Angeles Times,* pp. A3, A20.
Peterson, J.(2001, October 28). Welfare reform faces softening economy. *Los Angeles Times,* p. A31.
Pierson, P. (1995). *Dismantling the welfare state? Reagan, Thatcher, and the politics of retrenchment.* Cambridge, UK: Cambridge University Press.
Pigeon, M., & Wray, L. R. (1999). Did the Clinton rising tide lift all boats? *Challenge, 42,* 14-33.
Piven, F. F. (1999, Spring). What's really happening in South Carolina? *Social Policy, 29,* 34-37.
Piven, F. F., & Ellwood, D. (1996, July-August). Was welfare reform worthwhile? *The American Prospect, 27,* 14-15.
Pollin, R. (2000, May-June). Anatomy of Clintonomics. *New Left Review, 3 (New series),* 17-46.
Pryor, F. L., & Schaffer, D. L. (2000). *Who's not working and why: Employment, cognitive skills, wages, and the changing U.S. labor market.* Cambridge, UK: Cambridge University Press.
Reagan, R. (1988). Address before a joint session of Congress on the state of the union (February 8, 1986), in *Public papers of the presidents: Ronald Reagan, Book I.* DC: GPO.
Reich, R.B. (1997). *Locked in the cabinet.* NY: Alfred A. Knopf.
Ricketts, E. R., & Sawhill, I. V. (1988). Defining and measuring the underclass. *Journal of Policy Analysis and Management, 7,* 316-325.
Rivera, C. (2001, August 23). 5 years later, welfare reform draws fire from recipients and advocates. *Los Angeles Times,* p. B3.
Rosenblatt, R. A. (1996, June 8). Economic surge adds 348,000 jobs to U.S. work force. *Los Angeles Times,* pp. A1, A13.
Shriver, J. (2001, November 21). U.S. tech firms abusing visa program, critics say. *Los Angeles Times,* pp. A1, A29.
Silverstein, S. (1998, July 30). Missing the boom-time bandwagon. *Los Angeles Times,* pp. A1, A16.
Silverstein, S. (2000, June 3). Jump in jobless rate spurs rally in Nasdaq, Dow. *Los Angeles Times,* pp. A1, A14.
Simon, S. (2001, December 30). Welfare reform offers paradox. *Los Angeles Times,* p. A22.
Starr, A. (2000, May 22). Chipping away at the uninsured. *The American Prospect, 11,* 18-19.
States lag in promoting responsible dads as social norm. (1999, Summer). *News & Issues, 9* (National Center for Children in Poverty), 1-2.
Thurow, L. (1996, March-April). The crusade that's killing prosperity. *The American Prospect, 25,* 54-59.
Tonelson, A. (2000). *The race to the bottom: Why a worldwide worker surplus and uncontrolled free trade are sinking American living standards.* Boulder, CO: Westview Press.

Twentieth Century Fund (1998). *The basics: Social Security reform.* NY: Century Foundation Press.

Uchitelle, L. (2000, March 26). Companies try dipping deeper into the labor poor. *New York Times*, Section 1, pp. 1, 26.

U.S. Bureau of the Census (2001). *Poverty in the United States, 2000.* DC: GPO.

U.S. Congress (1996, August 22). Public Law 104-193. DC: GPO.

U.S. Department of Commerce, Bureau of Economic Analysis. Gross domestic product, in current dollars and in chained (1996) dollars, at http://www.bea.doc.gov/bea/dn/gdplev.htm.

Veith, W. (2001, December 8). Layoffs push jobless rate to 6-year high. *Los Angeles Times*, pp. C1, C3.

Walsh, M.W. (2000, January 19). Boom time a bad time for the poorest, study finds. *Los Angeles Times*, pp. A1, A12.

Western, B. (2001, Spring). Incarceration, unemployment, and inequality. *Focus 21*, 32-36.

Political Promises for Welfare Reform

Elizabeth A. Segal
Keith M. Kilty

SUMMARY. Public debate by policymakers prior to the passage of the PRWORA reflected a common set of attitudes and beliefs of those in power about public assistance and the poor. The power of their language to shape and inform policy is significant in our society. Those who hold power use language to mold and rationalize public policies. From a critical theory perspective, examination of the use of language by those in power to set norms, disempower, and marginalize those people who are nondominant is vital to effect social change. This research critically examines the speeches given on the floor of the House of Representatives prior to the final vote of PRWORA on July 31, 1996, to identify the power of language. Findings reveal that the content of the speeches reflects maintenance of the status quo and continued marginalization of the poor, particularly women. *[Article copies available for a fee from The Haworth Document Delivery Service: 1-800-HAWORTH. E-mail address: <docdelivery@haworthpress.com> Website: <http://www.HaworthPress.com> © 2003 by The Haworth Press, Inc. All rights reserved.]*

KEYWORDS. Political discourse, critical discourse analysis, power, welfare reform, women and public assistance, marginalization

---

Elizabeth A. Segal is Professor, School of Social Work, Arizona State University, Box 871802, Tempe, AZ 85287-1802.
Keith M. Kilty is Professor, College of Social Work, Ohio State University, 1947 College Road, Columbus, OH 43210.

[Haworth co-indexing entry note]: "Political Promises for Welfare Reform." Segal, Elizabeth A., and Keith M. Kilty. Co-published simultaneously in *Journal of Poverty* (The Haworth Press, Inc.) Vol. 7, No. 1/2, 2003, pp. 51-67; and: *Rediscovering the Other America: The Continuing Crisis of Poverty and Inequality in the United States* (ed: Keith M. Kilty, and Elizabeth A. Segal) The Haworth Press, Inc., 2003, pp. 51-67. Single or multiple copies of this article are available for a fee from The Haworth Document Delivery Service [1-800-HAWORTH, 9:00 a.m. - 5:00 p.m. (EST). E-mail address: docdelivery@haworthpress.com].

In his first run for the presidency, Bill Clinton made a campaign promise to "end welfare as we know it." Four years later, he had succeeded in achieving that promise when he signed the Personal Responsibility and Work Opportunity Reconciliation Act (PRWORA) in 1996. While Clinton may have made "welfare reform" a cornerstone of his campaign, he was certainly not alone in calling for change. The public outcry by policymakers for changing welfare prior to the passage of the PRWORA reflected a common set of attitudes and beliefs of those in power about public assistance and the poor. The power of their language to shape and inform policy is significant in our society. Those who hold power use language to mold and rationalize public policies. They have access to public forums, including the mass media, where they can express their beliefs and inform public opinion.

From a critical theory perspective, as demonstrated in the works of Michel Foucault (1972), Jurgen Habermas (1971) and Paulo Freire (1990), examination of the use of language by those in power to set norms, disempower, and marginalize those people who are nondominant is vital to effect social change. Analysis based on critical theory creates understanding of the balance of power, particularly as it relates to such social forces as gender, race, and class. This understanding is essential in order to generate praxis, i.e., social change and the means to advocate for a more egalitarian society.

This research critically examines the speeches given on the floor of the House of Representatives prior to the final vote of PRWORA on July 31, 1996. While numerous Congressional sessions and hearings covered welfare reform, the discussions on that day pertained to the actual legislation that became law. It is important to recognize that these speeches represent what policymakers are prepared to state publicly, rather than their private beliefs, attitudes, and ideologies. Therefore, examining the speeches using critical discourse analysis demonstrates the power of language to set norms, maintain the status quo, and oppress already-marginalized groups.

RELEVANT LITERATURE

Forty years ago, Michael Harrington (1962) made a remarkable discovery in this land of plenty: there was also poverty—or what he called "The Invisible Land." Based on his calculations, there were some 50 million poor in the United States. At that time, there was no official definition of poverty, nor was there much concern about those who were still poor in this country. The U.S. had emerged from World War II as the dominant economic and military power in the world, recovered from the terrible days of the Great Depression. Harrington's *The Other America* is often credited with raising public consciousness, especially that of policy-makers, about poverty in the midst of affluence and with being a major impetus behind President Lyndon Johnson's "War on Poverty" (Karger & Stoesz, 2002). The rhetoric about poverty and welfare in the 1960s, then, was very different from that of the 1980s and 1990s.

Poverty in the U.S., as in most societies, is nothing new. Whether recognized or not, it has certainly always existed here. Unfortunately, concern about poverty often disappears from the public scene, only to be rediscovered periodically. When we founded the *Journal of Poverty: Innovations on Social, Political & Economic Inequalities* in 1997, we dedicated it to the memories of three "pioneers in the continuing rediscovery of poverty and inequality": Frederick Douglass (1818-1895), Jane Addams (1865-1930), and Michael Harrington (1928-1990). The lives of those individuals span most of the existence of the country itself, reflecting the fact that progressives have struggled to raise awareness about and to change the conditions of the oppressed.

Unfortunately, even when poverty and the poor are acknowledged, public sentiments often depict the poor themselves as the main cause of their condition (Kilty & Segal, 1996). Throughout the history of this country, including the colonial era, the poor have been identified in terms of being "deserving" or "undeserving" of assistance (Gordon, 1994; Katz, 1989). This notion of who is deserving or undeserving is not only a popular and political conception but also one that is reflected in the writings of "liberal" social scientists, such as William Julius Wilson, who titled his 1987 book *The Truly Disadvantaged*. Yet the notion that people are poor because of immoral behavior and ignorance can be traced to the early nineteenth century writings of Thomas Malthus (Kilty & Segal, 1996). For at least the last two centuries, then, some social critics have identified the personal failings of the poor as the "true" cause of their poverty. In fact, the political rhetoric of the late twentieth century was much the same as that of the late nineteenth century when urban slums emerged due to the demands of industrialization and the poor were characterized as the "dangerous classes" (Coontz, 1992).

Clearly, then, the impetus for welfare reform in the early 1990s was nothing new. Opponents of the federal efforts to provide public assistance for poor women and children were numerous from the first passage of the program originally titled Aid to Dependent Children in 1935. Historical changes included expansions and contractions for sixty years. By the 1990s, the program was known as Aid to Families with Dependent Children (AFDC) and included among its provisions coverage of single-parent families for unlimited time as long as the families fell below the income eligibility level. This status as an entitlement program was cited as creating lifetime dependency and became the alleged strong rationale for reexamining the program. Then President Clinton made his famous remark to "end welfare as we know it," and Congress complied.

Many argue that the rationale for dismantling the program was far different from concern with dependency:

> Virtually all the ills afflicting American society are being attributed to single-mother families. Out-of-wedlock births have been blamed for the "breakdown of the family," as well as for the crime rate, drug and alcohol addiction, poverty, illiteracy, homelessness, poor school performance, and the rending of the social fabric. The labeling of some citizens as "dependent"–that is, dependent on social welfare programs rather than on spouses, parents, or other family members, or on other, more acceptable federal programs–has been used indiscriminately to discredit an entire group of women and children without regard to their character or their specific work and family history. (Sidel, 1996, p. 491)

The reasoning for welfare reform was that if single mothers could be put to work, then these problems would be solved. Although decades of research had failed to demonstrate the link between women's marital or childbearing status and the use of public assistance, the belief in that link became the impetus and rationale for changing the law (Abramovitz, 1996). As stated in the legislation, almost 90% of the children receiving AFDC were living in homes where no father was present. The assumption of policymakers was that if single women became married, the problem of welfare would be solved. These assumptions are evident in the provisions of the bill. The law cites four purposes: (a) to care for needy children in their own homes; (b) to end the dependence on government benefits of needy parents by promoting jobs, work, and marriage; (c) to prevent and reduce the incidence of out-of-wedlock pregnancies; and (d) to encourage the formation and maintenance of two-parent families (P.L. 104-193, section 401). The emphasis on marriage for single women and childbearing within marriage steep this legislation in the context of gender. Nowhere does the legislation address poverty as a structural concern or societal economic conditions as a context for public assistance.

Other factors related to poverty and welfare use have also been ignored by policymakers. Domestic violence can be found in about 6% of American households, yet 20% to 30% of women receiving public assistance are reported to be current victims (Raphael, 2000). And these numbers may be lower than the reality as violence in the home is often underreported. Why has the link between domestic violence and poverty been ignored?

> The existence of domestic violence makes the conservatives' mandatory work/"tough love" approach both ineffective and inappropriately harsh, with the potential for causing more violence. "Culture of poverty" theories, holding that welfare dependence or living in persistent poverty has sapped low-income persons' energy, causing depression, apathy, and helplessness, for which mandatory work is seen as the necessary antidote, crumble when confronted with a family problem such as domestic violence that cannot be remedied by mandatory work. (Raphael, 2000, p. 7)

Changing the labor market, raising wages, and improving child care, while worthy efforts, will not help women whose partners will not let them work or undermine their efforts to work through intimidation and violence. Thus, attention to domestic violence becomes the first step in "welfare reform" for up to possibly one-third of the women receiving public assistance. This fact suggests that debate surrounding welfare reform should also include debate about the ways to address domestic violence.

The link between race and ethnicity and poverty is also crucial to understanding the context of poverty in this country. In counts of poverty, the proportion of people of color who are impoverished is greater than that of the dominant white population (Dalaker, 2001). While female-headed families are more susceptible to poverty due in part to gender bias, for female-headed African American families, the rate is more than twice as high as for white female-headed families, 35% compared to 17%. Among the lowest rates of poverty are for married couple families, with white families recording 3.3% in poverty. Yet for nondominant families, the rate is 6.1% for African American families and 14.1% for Latino families. To ignore race and ethnicity in discussions of poverty is to miss a significant historical correlation.

The pervading sense that all previous efforts at eradicating poverty had failed further fueled the debate. This perception was strong, in spite of evidence to the contrary. Following the creation of anti-poverty programs, poverty in America decreased. While the average poverty rate in the 1960s was over 17.5%, it had decreased to less than 11.8% in the 1970s.

Even after cutbacks during the 1980s, the poverty rate averaged 13.75% during the 1990s, lower than before the War on Poverty (authors' calculations based on data in Dalaker, 2001). Government supports continue to be powerful in reducing poverty. According to a report from the Center on Budget and Policy Priorities, government assistance kept some 27 million poor, disabled, and elderly individuals above the poverty threshold, while the number of children in households below the poverty line fell from 24% to 16% after the receipt of public aid in 1995 (*Dollars and Sense*, 1997). Largely because of the State Children's Health Insurance Program (SCHIP), the number of children without health insurance in 2001 was 10.8%, compared to 13.9% in 1997 (Carter, 2002). Perhaps the most successful government anti-poverty is the old-age pension part of Social Security. In 1959, the poverty rate for the elderly was 35.2%, compared to 9.7% in 1999 (Karger & Stoesz, 2002). In fact, the Social Security Administration (2001) estimates that without Social Security benefits, the poverty rate for the elderly in 1999 would have been 48%. Nevertheless, many argued that reform was needed because all previous programs failed and had created a destructive dependency.

METHODOLOGY

Postmodern theory exhorts social scientists to examine the social order from the multiple perspectives of class, race, gender, and other identities (Agger, 1991). Critical theory takes that perspective a step further. Critical theory advocates understanding of oppression based on these identities and how those in power use these identities to disempower. Furthermore, critical theory calls for using understanding of oppression from the perspectives of class, race, gender and other identities to act as a catalyst for transforming society (Fay, 1987).

Using critical theory in research attempts "to describe the way media, political, educational, and other sociocultural productions coercively manipulate citizens to adopt oppressive meanings" (Kincheloe & McLaren, 2000, p. 283). This research combines critical theory with discourse analysis. Foucault's (1972) work linking discourse and power serves as part of the theoretical underpinning for this research. Discourse, power and knowledge are all intertwined. Political discourse, the domain of this research, has the force to influence and construct social meanings. Critical discourse analysis (CDA) is the methodology that combines critical theory with discourse analysis (Titscher, Meyer, Wodak, & Vetter, 2000). It is politically involved research that identifies power in discourse, power over discourse, and how society and culture are shaped by discourse.

CDA focuses on written text, and emphasizes both the details of the actual text and the political aspects of discourse: "The main purpose of critical discourse analysis is to understand how people are manipulated by public discourse and thereby subjected to abuses of power [and] . . . how public discourse often serves the interests of powerful forces over those of the less privileged" (Huckin, 2002, p. 158 & 159). This analysis of the discourse surrounding passage of the PRWORA employs the techniques of critical discourse analysis.

The sample chosen for analysis consisted of the texts delivered through speeches given on the floor of the House of Representatives preceding the final vote on PRWORA. These texts were chosen for several reasons. The House typically limits speeches to under three minutes, allowing for numerous perspectives to be delivered during debate. While over the year there were many debates on the merits of welfare reform, this analysis is concerned with what actually became law. Thus, the debates centered on the final version are most relevant and were therefore chosen as the texts of study. All the speeches that were delivered in person in the House of Representatives on July 31, 1996 immediately preceding the final vote on PRWORA were examined. Following the general steps of content analysis, frequency of themes or dimensions was assessed (Hansen, Cottle, Negrine, & Newbold, 1998). Three emergent themes were identified:

1. The view of the problem and why reform is needed;
2. The goal of the effort at welfare reform; and
3. The view of the pending legislation before the House.

Using a framework for CDA (Fairclough, 2001) emphasizing linguistic or semiotic analysis included: analysis of whole-text language, organization, combination of clauses, words, connotations, and collocations to detect meanings, ideologies, moods and norms. The research also employed discourse analysis techniques influenced by Foucault's theories that included looking for evidence of interrelationships, examining discursive strategies used, looking for absences and silences, and finally considering the context of the discourse (Carabine, 2000). Analysis also included quantitative methods based in content analysis to record the frequency of words and phrases used and the concerns raised. In keeping with CDA, the data were assessed with attention

FINDINGS

On July 31, 1996, 44 members of the House of Representatives took the floor to speak on pending welfare reform legislation (*Congressional Record*, 1996). The composition of those who spoke was not reflective of the total House membership. Of those 44 who chose to speak that day, 68% were males (n = 30) and 32% were females (n = 14) compared to the overall membership of 89% male and 11% female (see Table 1). The speakers tended to be against the bill more than the overall membership, with 36% of the speakers voting against the measure versus 23% of the overall membership (see Table 2). Women speakers voted similarly to women members in general, while 30% (n = 9) of the male speakers were opposed to the legislation compared to 21% (n = 80) of all the men in the House (see Table 3). For the House as a whole, 30% (14 out of 46) of the female members spoke that day while only 8% (30 out of 388) of the males took to the floor. In summary, those who chose to speak tended to represent opposition to the bill, were more likely to be Democrats, and were more likely to be women.

Emergent Themes

Speakers stressed three major areas in their speeches. They referred to the problem of welfare, the goal of changing the current system, and their assessments of the legislation before them. These three emergent themes dominated the debate.

TABLE 1. Comparison of Speakers and Overall House Membership

	Speakers (n = 44)	House as whole (n = 435)
Male	30 (68%)	389 (89%)
Female	14 (32%)	46 (11%)
Democrats	26 (59%)	204 (47%)
Republicans	18 (41%)	230 (53%)
Independents		1

TABLE 2. Votes on Welfare Reform

	Speakers (n = 44)	House as whole (n = 435)
Voted yes	28 (64%)	328 (76%)
Voted no	16 (36%)	101 (23%)
Did not vote		6 (1%)

View of the Problem and Why Reform Is Needed

The general sense that something was wrong and change was needed was shared by those who favored the bill as well as by those who opposed it. For example, one of those who spoke against the bill stated, "The welfare system does not work for the welfare recipients and for the taxpayers." While there was general agreement that something needed to be done, the precipitating factors varied. Some cited broad statements such as welfare was "a system that is broken" and "we have a failed welfare system." A strong sentiment emerged concerning dependency and the need to establish self-sufficiency:

> This goes a long way toward reforming our broken welfare system as we return the system to its original purpose–a temporary safety net, not a way of life.

There was a feeling that "no one should get something for nothing" and that the "current system does not meet the American values of work, opportunity, responsibility, and family." Even religion was eluded to:

> It is a sin not to help someone who genuinely, truly needs that help through no fault of their own, but it is also a sin to help people who do not need help. So this bill is going to encourage that personal responsibility that we are all so proud of and give people their dignity back.

The concerns raised as to why the legislation was needed were numerous. Reading through all the speeches revealed 23 different concerns. The two most commonly cited reasons were the need for individual responsibility and work requirements. Table 4 lists concerns raised by at least four different members. While children were a concern, they were brought up by those who opposed the bill, citing the lack of help the legislation would

TABLE 3. Votes on Welfare Reform by Gender

Women	Speakers (n = 14)	House as whole (n = 46)
Voted yes	7 (50%)	25 (54%)
Voted no	7 (50%)	21 (46%)
Men	Speakers (n = 30)	House as whole (n = 388)
Voted yes	21 (70%)	308 (79%)
Voted no	9 (30%)	80 (21%)

bring to the care of children. Noting absences and silences, topics never mentioned included substance abuse and neighborhood violence, correlates of poverty. Domestic violence was raised by one person, and that was to point out that the legislation ignored that issue. Education and training, historically touted as a way to self-sufficiency, was mentioned by only three speakers. Child care, another barrier for poor single parents, was mentioned by only three speakers. Poverty itself, while mentioned somewhere in the speech of 11 speakers, was not identified as a structural condition to be addressed. Rather, seven of those who mentioned it voted against the bill and raised concerns that the legislation itself would increase poverty. Only one speaker talked about poverty as a larger issue by stressing, "We must make sure that reform reduces poverty, not bashes poor people." The other four either saw a culture of poverty that needed to be addressed or the failure of the War on Poverty.

While most speakers limited themselves to general statements and beliefs, one cited as the problem the War on Poverty itself, and made a statement that data, as cited earlier in this paper, refute:

> Some 31 years [after launching the War on Poverty in 1965] poverty in America has worsened.

Thus, the dominant view of the problem was personal dependency and the lack of individual responsibility which must be instilled through required work. Absent were structural concerns and poverty as a social problem.

Goal of the Legislative Effort

The goals stated by the speakers reflected the concerns cited above. Personal responsibility on the part of recipients was a recurring theme:

TABLE 4. Concerns Raised Regarding Welfare Reform

	Frequency cited
Self reliance/individual responsibility Personal responsibility	9
Work requirements	9
State flexibility	8
Children	8
Fraud and abuse	5
Medical coverage	5
Get something for nothing/fairness to taxpayers	5
Child support enforcement improved	5
Out-of-wedlock births	4

> Welfare should not encourage, it should discourage destructive personal behavior that contributes so clearly not only to welfare dependence but to a host of social problems.
>
> Individuals must accept the responsibility of working and providing for their families.

New legislation was needed so that those who are recipients are not getting something for nothing. One legislator was pleased the bill "addresses the fundamental fairness issue in American society, and that is the resentment of working individuals toward able-bodied individuals who refuse to get off the dole." Some goals were vague, such as "solve the problems of the poor." Other goals were patriotic and symbolic, such as "reclaim our neighborhoods and help America" and "restore the work ethic." Many used poetic-sounding statements to state their goals. Collocation, juxtaposing words for impact, was used by several legislators. Moving from "a welfare check to a paycheck" and from a "caretaking society to a caring society" evoked strong images of policymakers making a bad system a good system. Other phrase collocations contrasted bad, those receiving welfare, versus good, those working independently:

- "Passive acceptance of a welfare check" versus "active earning of a paycheck."
- "Way of life" versus "safety net."
- "Lifetime of handouts" versus "temporary assistance."
- "A system that hurts people" versus "helping people to help themselves."

Contrasts were used to emphasize the dysfunction of the current system and its recipients and how the new legislation would restore function to the system and those who followed the new order.

Finally, there was the sense that new legislation would curb dysfunctional behaviors, particularly out-of-wedlock births:

> It addresses the problem of welfare dependency and welfare pathology in this country, which has led to soaring rates of family disintegration, illegitimacy in American society, and the other consequences, like youth crime.

View of the Legislation

As would be expected, those who voted for the bill saw the legislation as historical and an improvement over the current system. Numerous legislators considered the bill a "remarkable accomplishment" and "true welfare reform" as opposed to previous efforts that had failed to solve the problem. The extent of success was seen as far-reaching, creating an "independence day for welfare recipients" and "really reforming and empowering the states to be creative in solving their own problem and it will help end the cycle of dependency and poverty." The legislators were proud of themselves and felt they had created a "bill that shows good judgment by government."

For those opposed to the legislation, the discourse was full of concern and warnings:

> This legislation will not ensure families can live on jobs they get [or] that they will earn livable wage.

One of the strongest opposition voices cited the legislation as a

> deadly and Draconian piece of garbage which will do nothing to reform the conditions of poverty and unemployment suffered by our nation's most vulnerable.

And still another viewed it as

> dangerous and unrealistic; does not create jobs; federal cuts have already put people out on the street.

There was a feeling among opponents that the passage of welfare reform was politically expedient: "Scapegoating children is politically popular this year." As another stated:

> So when you look at it, this is a big political victory. The Democrats are happy in the White House. The Republicans are happy because they made him do it. The Governors are happy. They begged for the opportunity to do it their way after all. They are closer to the problem. And the only losers we have now are the kids.

IMPLICATIONS

Some points were clear from the words speakers chose to use. Self-sufficiency and personal responsibility were mentioned frequently, reinforcing the purpose of the PRWORA, as clearly stated in its title. Other implications were noticeable in the absence of being spoken. Silences can be as powerful as those words that are spoken. That structural poverty was not addressed reflects the lack of concern for eradicating poverty. That there was no mention of substance abuse and only one complaint about ignoring domestic violence attests to the lack of understanding or acceptance of larger social issues that correlate with poverty.

Gender was missing from the debate. Those who favored the legislation rarely identified adult recipients as women, although the vast majority of adult recipients are female. Terms used to identify those receiving public assistance were general, such as "welfare beneficiaries" or "welfare recipients" and as a family unit such as "disadvantaged families" or "welfare families." General references were made to "our Nation's low-income citizens." In comparison, identification of adult recipients as women and mothers did occur among the speeches of those in opposition.

"What if a mother on welfare cannot find a job?" was followed by concern about child care, typically the responsibility of women. Another complained, "This bill does nothing to train mothers for work." For those who supported this legislation, the fact that the roles of women such as child-rearing and birth and limitations for economic achievement based on gender are very real aspects of life for poor women went unmentioned. This silence means either lack of knowledge, or that those who fail to speak of gender do not accept it as part of the problem. Also, while almost 90% of the members of the House were male, 96% of the adult recipients of AFDC were female (Administration for Children and Families, 1995). That almost 80% of the men in the House voted to support the legislation, compared to 54% of the women, further demonstrates the gender imbalance. This unwillingness to speak of gender is true not only of politicians. The same ostensibly neutral (and therefore "objective") language used to identify welfare recipients is common in social science evaluations of welfare reform programs (Nelson, 2002).

Where gender does become an issue is in terms of the beliefs about deviant behavior. This legislation is clear that out-of-wedlock childbirth, lack of marriage, and personal responsibility are the problems. Low wages, corporate downsizing, globalization, lack of education and training, difficulty in being a single parent, inadequate child care, and insufficient benefits were not articulated concerns. While this may not be surprising, it is revealing. The words used by those in authority positions contribute greatly to the public consciousness. When elected officials in power neglect to acknowledge the true conditions of those who are disempowered and marginalized, then the power imbalance remains. By ignoring the gender reality for poor women, those in the majority, the supporters, reinforce the status quo that prevents women from gaining access to economic resources. This is precisely the evidence of the power of discourse to shape society.

Race and ethnicity are never mentioned. Completely ignoring the fact that a disproportionate number of the recipients of AFDC are people of color silences the role of race and ethnicity in the context of poverty. The assumption that personal responsibility is the key allows policymakers to ignore the realities that racism can and does impede employability and access to opportunity. This silence conveys the message that those in power do not consider race or ethnicity relevant, and, therefore, neither should the rest of society.

Class is another silence. Contextually it is noteworthy that members of Congress received an annual base pay of $141,300 in 2000 compared to the median household income that year of $42,148 (DeNavas-Walt,

Cleveland, & Roemer, 2001). Many members of Congress have income from other sources, and left very lucrative professions from which they amassed savings and investments. Most likely few, if any, experienced poverty while raising children, by definition the condition of every family receiving AFDC. In fact, most members of Congress have household incomes that place them in the top 5% of the U.S. population.

CONCLUSION

The fact that the two most prevalent concerns voiced by policymakers were the need for individual responsibility and work requirements sums up the intended impact of PRWORA. Poor women must be responsible for their and their children's well-being and they must do so through work. The irony that many of the legislators who promoted that position also advocated family values and creation of homes where parents are available to their children, seemed lost. The idea that a single mother can work full-time and earn enough to support herself and her children, and also have time to create a safe, nurturing, and stimulating environment in which to raise children was left unspoken. Maybe it was unspoken because it is impossible.

Ann Withorn (1996), who has interviewed many women who received public assistance, summed up the problem between political discourse and reality:

> Welfare is not, and should not be regarded as the worst thing that can happen to a poor woman. Life with an abusive partner, a job without adequate health benefits, insecure child care arrangements, lack of income, and humiliating bureaucratic harassment are all worse. (p. 508)

Much that is important to those who live in poverty and those who work with people living in poverty was never addressed. The impact of race and ethnicity, gender and class, individually and collectively, were never mentioned. Structural reasons for poverty were not addressed. Why?

> With six years' hindsight, it's hard to fathom why no one, back in 1996, seems to have thought ahead to a time when jobs would be in short supply and millions might sorely need cash assistance. (Ehrenreich & Piven, 2002, p. 41)

The answer to that is because, with the insight of critical theory, to raise those concerns would question the status quo. And to question the status quo would mean that those in power would have to take responsibility, as would society at large.

Critical discourse analysis reveals that those in power were intent on maintaining the status quo. The praxis drawn from this research is the need for advocates to give voice to the impact of race, gender and class on public assistance. The glaring discrepancies in race, gender, and class between those crafting welfare reform and those subject to the policy must be illuminated. The silences and absences within public welfare debates must be identified so that true reform can occur.

REFERENCES

Abramovitz, M. (1996). *Under attack: Fighting back: Women and welfare in the United States*. New York: Monthly Review Press.

Administration for Children and Families. (1995). *Characteristics and financial circumstances of AFDC recipients*. Washington, DC: U.S. Department of Health and Human Services.

Agger, B. (1991). *A critical theory of public life: Knowledge, discourse, and politics in an age of decline*. New York: The Falmer Press.

Carter, J. (2002). "More children have coverage, study says." *Columbus Dispatch*, June 15, A5.

Congressional Record. (1996). Volume 142, number 115, pp. H9403-9415.

Coontz, S. (1992). *The way we never were: American families and the nostalgia trap*. New York: Basic.

Dalaker, J. (2001). *Poverty in the United States: 2000*. Current Populations Reports, Series P60-214. Washington, DC: U.S. Government Printing Office.

DeNavas-Walt, C. Cleveland, R. W., & Roemer, M. I. (2001). Money income in the United States: 2000. P60-213. Washington, DC: U.S. Government Printing Office.

Dollars & Sense. (1997). "Poverty: Nostalgia for half-hearted programs." *Dollars & Sense*, January/February, 5.

Ehrenreich, B. & Piven, F. F. (2002). Without a safety net. *Mother Jones*, May/June, pp. 35-41.

Fay, B. (1987). *Critical social science*. Ithaca, NY: Cornell University Press.

Foucault, M. (1972). *The archeology of knowledge and the discourse of language*. New York: Random House.

Freire, P. (1990). *Pedagogy of the oppressed*. New York: Continuum.

Gordon, L. (1994). *Pitied but not entitled: Single mothers and the history of welfare*. Cambridge, MA: Harvard University Press.

Habermas, J. (1971). *Knowledge and human interests*. Boston: Beacon Press.

Hansen, A., Cottle, S. Negrine, R. & Newbold, C. (1998). *Mass communication research methods*. London: Macmillan Press Ltd.

Harrington, M. (1962). *The Other America: Poverty in the United States.* New York: Macmillan.
Huckin, T. (2002). Critical discourse analysis and the discourse of condescension. In E. Barton & G. Stygall (eds.). *Discourse studies in composition,* pp. 155-176. Cresskill, New Jersey: Hampton Press, Inc.
Karger, H. J. & Stoesz, D. (2002). American social welfare policy: A pluralist approach. (4th ed.). Boston: Allyn and Bacon.
Katz, M. B. (1989). *The undeserving poor: From the war on poverty to the war on welfare.* New York: Pantheon.
Kilty, K. M. & Segal, E. A. (1996). "Genetics and biological determinism: Scientific breakthrough or blaming the victim revisited?" *Humanity & Society, 20,* 3, 90-110.
Kincheloe, J. L. & McLaren, P. (2000). Rethinking critical theory and qualitative research. In N.K. Denzin & Y.S. Lincoln (Eds.), *Handbook of qualitative research.* 2nd Ed., pp. 279-313. Thousand Oaks, CA: Sage.
Nelson, M. K. (2002). "Declaring welfare 'reform' a success: The role of applied social science." *Journal of Poverty: Innovations on Social, Political & Economic Inequalities, 6* (3), 1-27.
Raphael, J. (2000). *Saving Bernice: Battered women, welfare, and poverty.* Boston: Northeastern University Press.
Sidel, R. (1996). The enemy within: A commentary on the demonization of difference. *American Journal of Orthopsychiatry, 66,* 4, 490-495.
Social Security Administration. (2001). *Fast facts & figures about social security.* (SSA Publication No. 13-11785). Washington, DC: Social Security Administration.
Wilson, W. J. (1987). *The truly disadvantaged: The inner city, the underclass, and public policy.* Chicago: University of Chicago Press.
Withorn, A. (1996). "Why do they hate me so much?": A history of welfare and its abandonment in the United States. *American Journal of Orthopsychiatry, 66,* 4, 496-509.

The "Other America" After Welfare Reform: A View from the Nonprofit Sector

David Sommerfeld
Michael Reisch

SUMMARY. This article examines the experiences of private, nonprofit social service agencies and their role in the "social safety net" following the 1996 welfare reforms. Among other concerns, the research suggests that declining welfare rolls are not indicative of widespread poverty reduction and increased self-sufficiency, as many nonprofits, especially those providing emergency food and shelter services, have experienced increasing demands during this time period. On a positive note, the growing role of nonprofit advocacy work emerged as one mechanism for improving the popular and political response to those living in poverty or near poverty conditions. *[Article copies available for a fee from The Haworth Document Delivery Service: 1-800-HAWORTH. E-mail address: <docdelivery@haworthpress.com> Website: <http://www.HaworthPress.com> © 2003 by The Haworth Press, Inc. All rights reserved.]*

David Sommerfeld is a PhD student in the Joint Social Work and Sociology Doctoral Program at the University of Michigan, Ann Arbor, MI 48109 (E-mail: dsommerf@umich.edu).

Michael Reisch is Professor of Social Work, University of Michigan, Ann Arbor, MI 48109 (E-mail: mreisch@umich.edu). He has been involved in research, advocacy, policy analysis and community organizing in the areas of poverty and welfare for over thirty years.

The research for this paper was funded by a grant from the Nonprofit Sector Research Fund, Aspen Institute.

[Haworth co-indexing entry note]: "The 'Other America' After Welfare Reform: A View from the Nonprofit Sector." Sommerfeld, David, and Michael Reisch. Co-published simultaneously in *Journal of Poverty* (The Haworth Press, Inc.) Vol. 7, No. 1/2, 2003, pp. 69-95; and: *Rediscovering the Other America: The Continuing Crisis of Poverty and Inequality in the United States* (ed: Keith M. Kilty, and Elizabeth A. Segal) The Haworth Press, Inc., 2003, pp. 69-95. Single or multiple copies of this article are available for a fee from The Haworth Document Delivery Service [1-800-HAWORTH, 9:00 a.m. - 5:00 p.m. (EST). E-mail address: docdelivery@haworthpress.com].

KEYWORDS. Welfare reform, nonprofit organizations, social services, poverty, advocacy

INTRODUCTION

The Personal Responsibility and Work Opportunity Reconciliation Act (PRWORA) of 1996 significantly changed the structure as well as the substance of U.S. social policymaking through its replacement of the 60-year-old AFDC program with federal block grants to the states. This fundamental shift in the U.S. welfare state has prompted a proliferation of scholarly and pragmatic research endeavors. Most of the attention has focused either on the macro-level data regarding state and national caseload reductions or micro-level data concerning the characteristics of and outcomes for individual welfare recipients (Allen and Kirby, 2000). This bifurcation of the analyses misses a key component of the U.S. social welfare system, nonprofit human service organizations. These private, charitable organizations are specially situated to gauge the impact of welfare reform on the "other America" as many assist and serve the low-income populations previously and/or currently involved with the public welfare system. Clearly, a comprehensive assessment of welfare reform's effect on low income populations must incorporate the experiences of these organizations.

By devolving responsibility for welfare programs to states and localities, the PRWORA increased the role of the private sector and faith-based organizations in program implementation and service provision (Cnaan, Wineburg, and Boddie, 1999). The act affirmed the implicit and explicit partnership between government agencies and nonprofit human service organizations and made a range of services provided by nonprofits both more critical to clients' success and more complicated to access (Bloom, 1997; Burt, Pindus, and Capizzano, 2000). Two underlying assumptions of the 1996 PRWORA were that the majority of welfare recipients would find employment within the statutory time limits and that private, nonprofit organizations would have sufficient capacity to care for those still needing additional supports. The purpose of this study was to examine the experiences of nonprofit human service organizations during the past four years to assess the validity of the second assumption.

This paper presents key findings related to the impact of welfare reform on 90 Southeastern Michigan nonprofit organizations and the clients they serve. Utilizing qualitative and quantitative data from the survey and several focus groups, the paper explores the extent of changes produced by welfare reform between 1996-2000 on (1) the client populations served by these organizations; (2) program goals, objectives, and outcomes; (3) funding sources and amounts; (4) emerging patterns of inter-organizational relationships to address client needs; and (5) the relationship with governmental agencies. The results indicate how public policies are transforming the nature of nonprofit organizations at the community level and how such organizations are responding to these external forces to meet the changing demands of low-income populations. Therefore, PRWORA's "success" must be defined by more than declining welfare rolls since economic and social hardships persist and give some appearances of increasing among the populations served by the private, nonprofit sector organizations, even during the period of tremendous economic growth characterizing the mid and late 1990s.

REVIEW OF THE LITERATURE

Although policy makers have acknowledged the potential effects of welfare reform on private, nonprofit organizations (U.S. Senate, Committee on Labor and Human Resources, 1996), most research to date has focused on its impact on recipients (Michigan League for Human Services, 1998; Besharov, Germanis, and Rossi, 1997) or on public sector agencies (Carnochan and Austin, 1999). Few studies have examined nonprofits' role in implementing welfare reform or on the impact of policy change on the organizations themselves, particularly on those agencies that serve predominantly racial minority clients (Besharov, Germanis, and Rossi, 1997; Hassett and Austin, 1997; Johnson, 1998; Briggs, 1999; Raffel, 1998; Perlmutter, 1997; Riccio and Orenstein, 1996).

Several recent research projects, however, have analyzed the impact of the 1996 welfare reforms on nonprofit human service organizations. These studies have a common theme: the decrease in welfare caseloads does not provide an adequate measure of the "success" of welfare reform, particularly since nonprofit human service organizations have experienced greater demands for their services from clients with more complex needs during the past four years (Fink and Widom, 2001; Bischoff, 2001; DiPadova, 2000; Withorn, 1999; Eisenger, 1999). The reduction in state welfare caseloads appears to represent, in part, a shift to a greater reliance on the nonprofit sector for needed supports. The increased level of client demand is especially troubling in light of the fact that the U.S. experienced what some might refer to as "the best of times" due to the dramatic economic expansion of the 1990s.

Recent research also demonstrates that welfare reform will intensify the economic and social problems confronting low-income neighborhoods, with particularly deleterious effects on individuals and families most dependent on the services nonprofits provide (Albelda, 1998; Alexander, 1999; Kittay, 1998; Meyer and Cancian, 1998; Swigonski, 1996; Jencks, 1996). It remains to be seen whether the combination of sectarian and non-sectarian organizations can fill the gaps created by the reduction in public sector support. The research undertaken by this current project is critical for developing a greater understanding of nonprofit organizations and their enhanced role in our nation's social safety net.

WELFARE AND WELFARE REFORM IN MICHIGAN

The State of Michigan began significantly reforming welfare policies and programs in 1992, introducing a statewide initiative that shifted the emphasis of the state's welfare policies from entitlement to individual personal responsibility. Within this context, the federal welfare reforms of 1996 did not represent a completely new modus operandi for Michigan, but rather another step in a series of reforms. Therefore, nonprofits in Michigan have had more time than their counterparts in most other states to acclimate to the changes produced by welfare reform. It is important to note, therefore, the findings from our study may actually underestimate the actual impact of PRWORA as experienced by nonprofit organizations elsewhere, since this research project used 1996 as the baseline year of comparison.[1]

Additionally, while welfare caseloads have dropped significantly in Michigan and nationwide, there seems to be a greater concentration in urban communities. In 1999, 33% of the nation's welfare caseload resided in ten urban counties (including Wayne County, Michigan) as compared to 24% in 1994 (Allen and Kirby, 2000). Although poverty has declined in many communities, urban areas continue to have poverty rates twice that of their surrounding suburbs, 16% to 8%, respectively (U.S. Census Bureau, CPS 2000).

RESEARCH METHODOLOGY AND SAMPLE CHARACTERISTICS

During the spring and summer of 2000 the researchers developed a listing of 501c (3) organizations from Washtenaw and Wayne Counties that provided health or human services to potential TANF populations (young children and/or their caretakers) that were in operation at the time of the legislation's passage (see Table 1 for county characteristics). Based on these criteria, an initial sample of 215 organizations (84 in Washtenaw County and 131 in Wayne County) was developed. Further scrutiny reduced this sample to 201 agencies.

Of these organizations, eighty-two returned the survey questionnaire (35 from Washtenaw County and 47 from Wayne County), an initial response rate of 41%. In addition, three focus groups were conducted, two in Wayne County and one in Washtenaw County, involving 32 participants from 30 agencies. Eight of the organizations represented at the focus groups did not return a survey. Therefore, we were able to collect survey and/or focus group data from a total of 90 organizations, 45% of the sample.

TABLE 1. County Comparisons

	Wayne County	Washtenaw County
2000 Population	2,061,162	322,895
2000 Racial Composition		
% White	52%	77%
% African American	42%	12%
1997 Est. Poverty Rate	18.0%	8.7%
1997 Est. Child Poverty Rate	28.5%	12.0%
1997 Est. Median Household Inc	$35,357	$51,286
TANF Caseload - 4/00	31,593	1,088
TANF Rate/county resident 4/00	43 / 1000	10 / 1000
2000 TANF Racial Composition		
% White	14%	32%
% African American	81%	60%
Caseload Reduction 3/94 - 4/00 *	66%	69%

* National caseload reduction (1/94 - 12/99)   53%

Sources:
Michigan's Family Independence Agency
U.S. Census Bureau
U.S. Department of Health and Human Services

The questionnaire generated both quantitative and qualitative data related to the breadth and depth of change experienced by the community organizations. Five variables were used for comparative analysis: agency location, agency type/focus, budget size, and the proportions of racial minority and public assistance (PA) clients served by the agency. The characteristics of the participating organizations are listed in Table 2.[2]

Data Analysis and Limitations

Throughout this paper, findings are considered statistically significant if $p < .05$. For categorical analyses, independence was tested by computing chi-square and, where low cell frequencies determined, Fisher's Exact Test. Association between ordinal level data was determined by computing Kendall's Tau. Statistical tests include only the questionnaire respondents. Certain questions (noted in the tables and the text) were applicable to only a subset of the responding organizations. Additionally, not all respondents answered each question, so some questions are missing data from the full sample. The number of respondents for each question is listed in the text and on the tables. With the reduced N for certain questions, substantial proportional variations may fail to pass standard statistical significance levels of $p < .05$. Therefore, some of the findings are suggestive, but not statistically significant.

Throughout the period of PRWORA's implementation, a number of political and economic changes have contributed to an increasingly complex operating environment for nonprofits. Due to these multifaceted contextual influences, a note of caution may be warranted concerning the ability of respondents to identify correctly the "source" of the changes they reported. While acknowledging this difficulty, the researchers believe the survey's two-step question process of inquiring about changes between 1996 and 2000 for a specific area, such as budget size, and then asking whether any reported changes were due to changes in welfare policy reduces the likelihood of conflating changes in the general environment and those related specifically to welfare reform. Given the substantial variations in the responses to these two types of questions (i.e., general change as compared to changes related to welfare reform), we believe that respondents were able to make the distinction. Additionally, qualitative responses frequently provided the rationale for whether or not a change was attributable to welfare reform.

TABLE 2. Sample Characteristics–Organizations

	Total Sample	Wayne County	Washtenaw County
Revised Sample Size	n = 77	47	30
	n	\multicolumn{2}{c	}{Percentages}
Agency Type			
Community/Multi-Service	35	34	37
Advocacy/Info/Education	18	15	20
Mental Health/Substance Abuse	26	32	17
Emergency Assistance	22	19	27
	(n = 77)	(47)	(30)
Proportion – Racial Minority Clients*			
Less than 30%	24	9	50
Between 30 - 70%	31	23	43
Greater than 70%	45	68	7
	(n = 75)	(47)	(28)
Proportion – Public Assistance Clients			
Less than 30%	19	15	26
Between 30 - 70%	44	44	44
Greater than 70%	37	41	30
	(n = 73)	(46)	(27)
Annual Budget*			
$250,000 or less	24	13	41
Between $250,000 and $1 million	23	26	21
Greater than $1,000,000	53	61	38
	(n = 75)	(46)	(29)
Staff Size*			
Less than 10 employees	33	26	43
Between 10 and 50	31	25	40
More than 50	35	49	17
	(n = 77)	(47)	(30)

*Significant difference between Wayne and Washtenaw County (p < .05)

FINDINGS

Changes in Client Demand and Composition

One dominant issue expressed in the survey responses as well as the focus groups concerned the increase in client demand experienced by nonprofit organizations between 1996 and 2000. While considerable variation existed among respondents, the median change in the number of clients served during this period was an increase of 26%. The median change value was similar in both counties and among all size organizations, although substantial variation existed by organization type. (See Table 3.)

Multi-service/community-based organizations registered the greatest increase in clients served. In contrast, nearly half (46%) of the emergency service organizations indicated serving the same or fewer clients. On the surface, this simple finding appears to refute the argument that economic conditions for the poor are deteriorating and that nonprofit organizations are confronted with the need to shore up an eroding social safety net. The focus-group discussions, however, provided further insight into this issue.

Most of the organizations that provided emergency shelter commented that the limited number of beds they possess constrains the number of clients they can serve, regardless of how many individuals seek shelter. Several respondents commented that their agencies have been operating at full capacity throughout the entire period. In addition, emergency service providers reported that shelter residents are taking longer to find permanent housing. As a result, several shelters actually reported a decrease in clients served, even as demand increased or remained constant.

Changes also occurred in the proportion of clients served who receive public assistance (PA). Reflecting the overall decline in TANF welfare rolls, 77% of the organizations indicated serving either the same or a lower proportion of public assistance clients in 1999 as they did in 1996. This proportion was fairly consistent regardless of organization location, type, client demographics, or agency budget. Over one-third of the organizations reported at least a 10% decline, and only 16% indicated an increase of 10% or more. Organizations located in Wayne County were slightly more likely to indicate a decrease of at least 10% than those from Washtenaw County (41% vs. 27%). Over half (53%) of the emergency service organizations reported at least a 10% decline in the proportion of PA clients served and none reported an increase greater than 10%.

TABLE 3. Changes in Client Demand and Composition

	Total %	Location Wayne	Location Wash.	Organizational Type[#] Com.	Organizational Type[#] Adv/ Info	Organizational Type[#] MH/ SA	Organizational Type[#] Emg. Svcs	% Racial Min. Clnts. Low <30%	% Racial Min. Clnts. Med. 30-70	% Racial Min. Clnts. High >70%	% Public Asst. Clnts. Low <30%	% Public Asst. Clnts. Med. 30-70	% Public Asst. Clnts. High >70%	Annual Budget Low <$250K	Annual Budget Med.	Annual Budget High >$1M.
Median percent change in number of clients served between 1996 and 1999.[a] (n = 58)	26	29	25	45	16	25	23	25	39	27	25	25	33	25	31	29
Change in the ratio of PA vs. non-PA clients served between 1996 and 1999. (n = 61)																
Proportion reporting the same or a declining proportion of PA clients served.	77	77	77	67	64	82	93	81	88	68	85	76	74	85	65	81
Proportion reporting a greater than 10% *decrease* in PA clients served.	36	41	27	33	9	41	53	38	29	39	39	60	9	39	47	29
Proportion reporting a greater than 10% *increase* in PA clients served.	16	15	18	22	36	12	0	19	6	21	15	16	17	15	29	10

[a] All median *percent change* values represent *percent increases* given the widespread growth in the number of clients served.

[#] Com. = Community/Multi-Service;   Adv/Info = Advocacy/Info/Education;   MH/SA = Mental Health/Substance Abuse; and Emg. Svcs = Emergency Services

This finding provides some support for the assertion that declining welfare rolls do not necessarily reflect greater self-sufficiency among former recipients, as other studies have noted (Abramovitz, 2002; Withorn, 1999). In fact, numerous respondents commented that welfare reform has increased the number of clients they serve who are classified as "working poor." Their agencies have adjusted eligibility standards and program focus to accommodate this increase. Respondents also stated that some clients are earning more but are unable to keep up with cost of living increases and the additional expenses of maintaining a job. They noted that work requirements had particularly increased the level of stress among women, who are employed in "go-nowhere jobs."

The increased need for emergency services and other social supports for those who have been removed from the welfare rolls or those not eligible for public assistance represent a real challenge for the nonprofit sector. For example, one respondent commented that her organization ran a job-training program for people who had attempted but failed to meet the requirements of publicly funded programs. Thus, nonprofit sector activity has increased not only because of public-private partnerships to provide services, but also to support those individuals and families who have "fallen through the cracks" in publicly funded or administered programs.

Client Referrals

One factor contributing to increased client demand during the past four years has been the growth in the number of referrals received. Most (80%) of the agencies (n = 69) reported an increase in referrals, while only 7% reported a decline. Many of these referrals are for emergency services such as food and shelter. Factors cited for the increased number of referrals included the development of expanded provision through the use of collaboratives, overall increase in clients, the growth in the number of harder-to-serve clients who require a complex network of services, the decline in the number of service providers, the effects of funding cuts, and the impact of rising demand and stagnant or declining resources.

Duration of Client Contact

In addition to an increase in client demand, almost half (47%) of the respondents (n = 70) reported an increase in the duration of client contact during the past four years. This increase was particularly apparent among emergency assistance organizations (69% as compared to only 41% of other types of agencies), which have had to adjust to a greater demand for services as well as to longer or cyclical periods of client contact (p = .008). One respondent referred to "more repeat requests . . . from people trying hard but not able to get resources." Another respondent stated, "Clients are more difficult to serve than last year. We are working with the 'gut-bucket bottom' [the ones worst off]." The short-term orientation of programs means that these clients' "problems will never be addressed." Clients are "cycling" back for additional assistance and requiring more intensive/multiple services.

Changes in Agency Programs

In response to growing client demand and the increasingly complex nature of clients' problems, many agencies (77%; n = 74) reported the development of new programs or the expansion of existing services in such areas as employment training. Half of the respondents (n = 72) indicated that changes in welfare policies had affected the primary program activities of their agency. In focus groups, participants cited the shifting orientation toward work-related programs as the most important effect of welfare reform. (See Table 4.)

Given the transformation and expansion of service provision, nearly two-thirds (66%) of the respondents (n = 70) indicated that their agency's program *objectives* and over 70% of respondents (n = 67) indicated that their program *outcomes* had changed during the past four years. Agency size was positively associated with changes in both program objectives and program outcomes, with approximately 40% of small, 60% of medium, and slightly over 80% of large organizations indicating such changes.

As anticipated, the proportion of PA clients served was significantly associated with whether respondents related changes in program objectives and outcomes to welfare reform. For example, of those respondents who indicated changes in program *objectives* (n = 44), only 25% of those serving a small proportion of PA clients as compared to 50% of moderate and 81% of organizations serving a large proportion of PA clients indicated that welfare reform had affected program objectives (p = .007). A similar pattern was evident for program *outcomes*, with agencies serving higher proportions of public assistance organizations significantly more likely to indicate changes due to welfare reform. Additionally, most emergency service providers (70%) related changes in outcomes to welfare policy as compared to the other types of organizations (36%).

TABLE 4. Changes in Agency Programs

	Total %	Location Wayne	Location Wash.	Organizational Type # Com. Info	Organizational Type # Adv/ Info	Organizational Type # MH/ SA	Organizational Type # Emg. Svcs.	% Racial Min. Clnts. Low <30%	% Racial Min. Clnts. Med. 30-70	% Racial Min. Clnts. High >70%	% Public Asst. Clnts. Low <30%	% Public Asst. Clnts. Med. 30-70	% Public Asst. Clnts. High >70%	Annual Budget Low <$250K	Annual Budget Med.	Annual Budget High >$1M
Proportion reporting an increase in primary agency activities during the past four years. (n = 74)	77	77	78	76	67	70	94	77	82	76	77	74	85	72	71	84
Proportion reporting that changes in welfare policies altered their primary program activities. (n = 72)	50	57	39	60	27	45	56	31	41	69**	33	53	59	35	44	61
Proportion reporting changes in program *objectives* during the past four years. (n = 70)	66	71	56	79	50	55	71	56	68	71	64	68	64	39	60	81**
Proportion reporting changes in welfare policies affected program objectives. (n = 44) [a]	55	63	36	56	20	64	60	33	57	65	25	50	81**	20	44	66

Proportion reporting changes in program *outcomes* during the past four years. (n = 67)	70	74	63	75	60	70	69	63	79	73	62	80	69	40	67	83**
Proportion reporting that changes in welfare policies affected program outcomes. (n = 43) [b]	44	48	36	38	0	46	70	40	43	47	12	53 ^		50	40	46

* Significant linear association (p < .01)
^ Significant Chi-square difference (p < .05) exists when these two categories collapsed.
[a] Includes only organizations that indicated changes in program objectives
[b] Includes only organizations that indicated changes in program outcomes
Com. = Community/Multi-Service;   Adv/Info = Advocacy/Info/Education;   MH/SA = Mental Health/Substance Abuse;   and Emg. Svcs = Emergency Services

81

Need for Provision of Emergency Services

Respondents particularly noted the impact of policy changes on emergency services, such as the increased use of free meals and other food assistance programs. As providers in other cities have reported (Abramovitz, 2002; Abramovitz, 2000; DiPadova, 2000; Withorn, 1999), agencies operating food pantries are now overwhelmed. They have had to expand nutrition services and revise their methods of food distribution. One agency reported serving 785 people in its Sunday soup kitchen (an increase of ~300%). One respondent remarked "[c]lients track me down for food wherever they see me, even during non-working hours." Another noted that clients are now asking for food assistance for the entire month, not only for a few days before their welfare checks arrive.

The demand for emergency shelter has also increased dramatically. An agency executive stated "[w]alk-in centers are sometimes so crowded there is standing room only." Yet, while one organization added two programs for homeless people since the introduction of welfare reform, others reported having to reduce the number of clients served in shelters due to the increasing length of the average stay. They estimate that they are serving only about one-fourth the people who are in need. As a consequence of welfare reform, one respondent remarked, "[a]ll our fears were realized; there is an increased demand for services with no corresponding increase in funding."

Others commented on how their agencies had expanded services into new areas, had developed more individualized client programs, and had shifted their goals from "band-aid" approaches to long-term self-sufficiency. Some respondents, however, used the language of survival to describe their program outcomes. They spoke of filling the gaps created by welfare reform. Agencies are thus torn between meeting people's basic survival needs and helping them find and keep employment. One respondent stated, "[f]ewer people are getting back on their feet. They hop from one weak support system to another. [There is a] lack of permanency in their lives."

Welfare Policy and Agency Budgets

Over half of the agencies (n = 69) reported that welfare policy changes had affected the *size* of their budgets and slightly less than half, 45%, indicated that welfare policy changes had affected the *source* of their budgets. The most commonly cited reason for budget increases was service expansion. For both budget size and sources, the proportion of PA clients served was significantly associated with the prevalence and depth of impact related to changes in welfare policy. (See Table 5.)

Respondents' comments were equally divided among those that emphasized the relationship between service expansion and recent budget increases and those that described how their agencies are attempting to serve more clients with the same or decreased funding. Funding "success" appears to be a function of whether an organization provides services that correspond to the welfare-to-work orientation of PRWORA. For some, contracts with Michigan's Family Independence Agency (FIA) or other funding sources have resulted in substantially increased budgets over the past four years. However, others complained of the difficulties involved in obtaining available public sector funds and of increased competition for fewer public dollars. Organizations providing critical emergency services to low-income clients received no substantial increase in public funds, even though demand has increased significantly. These fiscal difficulties are compounded, some respondents said, by a decline in private donations "since the general public believes that we don't have a problem." One respondent remarked, "[t]he public's perception is that employment is up and everyone is working. That's not the reality and it's hard to get that message out."

In response to the budgetary implications of welfare reform, 21% of the organizations increased staff workloads or reduced the number of staff, 8% rationed their client services, and 8% eliminated some services entirely. Clearly, service provision for low-income clients has been compromised in certain organizations.

Inter-Organizational Activities

Given the importance of inter-organizational relationships within the contemporary social safety net, respondents were also queried about their activities with other organizations. (See Table 6.) The vast majority (84%) indicated voluntary participation in service provision collaboration and close to half (43%) were involved in service provision collaborations required by their funding sources. One potentially positive finding from the research concerned the proportion (64%) of organizations indicating involvement in advocacy/coalition work on behalf of their clients. This type of activity was especially common among Wayne County organizations (76%). Inter-organizational advocacy work is crucial for low-income populations and those comprising the "other America" since, in general, they frequently lack opportunities for

TABLE 5. Welfare Policy and Agency Budgets

	Total %	Location		Organizational Type #				% Racial Min. Clnts.			% Public Asst. Clnts.			Annual Budget		
		Wayne	Wash.	Com.	Adv/ Info	MH/ SA	Emg. Svcs.	Low <30%	Med. 30-70	High >70%	Low <30%	Med. 30-70	High >70%	Low <$250K	Med.	High >$1M.
Organizations reporting that changes in welfare policies had an impact on the *size* of the agency's budget. (n = 69)	52	60	41	42	46	60	63	35	43	69*	25	48	72**	41	47	61
Organizations reporting that changes in welfare policies had an impact on the *sources* of the agency's budget. (n = 69)	45	46	43	48	36	37	56	33	38	57	25	41	60*	35	47	50

* Significant linear association (p <= .05)
** Significant linear association (p <= .01)
\# Com. = Community/Multi-Service; Adv/Info = Advocacy/Info/Education; MH/SA = Mental Health/Substance Abuse; and Emg. Svcs = Emergency Services

TABLE 6. Purposes of Inter-Organizational Work

	Total %	Location Wayne	Location Wash.	Organizational Type # Com.	Organizational Type # Adv/Info	Organizational Type # MH/SA	Organizational Type # Emg. Svcs.	% Racial Min. Clnts. Low <30%	% Racial Min. Clnts. Med. 30-70	% Racial Min. Clnts. High >70%	% Public Asst. Clnts. Low <30%	% Public Asst. Clnts. Med. 30-70	% Public Asst. Clnts. High >70%	Annual Budget Low <$250K	Annual Budget Med.	Annual Budget High >$1M
Collaborations for service provision (voluntary) (n = 75)	84	85	83	85	75	90	82	77	96	82	86	84	89	77	83	90
Collaborations for service provision (required) (n = 75)	43	50	31	50	17	50	41	35	44	49	7	48	56**	6	28	64**
Advocacy/coalition work (n = 75)	64	76	45 ^^	54	58	70	77	59	52	76	50	61	78	47	61	74*
Training/technical assistance (n = 75)	48	63	24 ^^	39	58	50	53	24	44	67**	57	36	59	29	44	56
Information sharing (n = 75)	91	94	86	96	83	90	88	88	91	94	86	90	96	65	94	100**
Fundraising/ resource sharing (n = 75)	35	41	24	31	50	35	29	24	44	36	43	32	33	24	44	33

^^ Significant Chi-square difference (p <= .05)
* Significant linear association (p <= .05)
** Significant linear association (p <= .01)
# Com. = Community/Multi-Service; Adv/Info = Advocacy/Info/Education; MH/SA = Mental Health/Substance Abuse; and Emg. Svcs = Emergency Services

developing a strong political voice or even a positive, visible presence in mainstream culture. Therefore, advocacy through nonprofit organizations represents one mechanism for engaging the broader community, especially policy makers, in the struggle against poverty. Larger agencies were much more likely to engage in this type of advocacy or coalition work. Nearly three-fourths of large agencies reported such efforts, as compared with 61% of mid-size agencies and only 47% of small agencies (p = .05). According to the qualitative data collected, this may be explained by the fact that smaller agencies are "operating in survival mode." According to one respondent, this condition "prevents and inhibits efforts to organize and exert collective power."

Relationships with Governmental Agencies

Respondents were also asked about changes in their relationship to government agencies. Nearly two-thirds of the respondents (n = 71) indicated that accountability requirements had increased during the past four years. Although a majority of respondents reported increases in accountability requirements, only slightly over one-fourth of all respondents reported increased government controls. (See Table 7.)

Over half of the respondents (55%) reported increased client advocacy with government agencies during the previous four years. Multi-service agencies were more likely to report an increase in client advocacy (71%) than were emergency assistance (56%), advocacy organizations (55%), and mental health agencies (35%). Some respondents commented on the need to become an expert on FIA procedures and practices in order to effectively advocate for their clients, which further drains valuable staff time and resources. "I had to learn how to do the job of an FIA worker in order to work with the system enough to get things done. It was a difficult and time consuming process."

Although welfare policies have often generated increased organizational strain, less than one-fourth of the respondents reported that their relationships with government staff in such departments as the Family Independence Agency had become more adversarial. Agencies with large proportions of welfare clients were more than twice as likely to report increased adversarial relationships (35% vs. 17%). Interestingly, agencies from suburban Washtenaw County were almost twice as likely to indicate a more adversarial relationship than their urban Wayne County counterparts (32% vs. 17%). The discussion from the focus groups suggested an interpretation, such that Wayne County organizations already experienced a certain level of tension with government

TABLE 7. Relationship with Governmental Agencies

	Total	Location		Organizational Type #			% Racial Min. Clnts.			% Public Asst. Clnts.			Annual Budget		
	%	Wayne	Wash.	Com.	Adv/ Info	MH/ SA	Emg. Svcs.	Low <30%	Med. 30-70	High >70%	Low <30%	Med. 30-70	High >70%	Low <$250K	Med.	High >$1M.
Increased accountability/ reporting requirements (n = 71)	63	72	48^	79	36	80	38^	47	76	68	77	59	69	27	69	77**
Greater need for information or technical assistance (n = 71)	41	46	32	46	18	45	44	18	50^		23	38	58*	27	38	49
Needed assistance in interpreting legislative or regulatory changes (n = 71)	28	33	20	25	27	40	19	24	33	29	39	14	42^	27	25	31

TABLE 7 (continued)

	Total %	Location Wayne	Location Wash.	Organizational Type # Com.	Organizational Type # Adv/Info	Organizational Type # MH/SA	Organizational Type # Emg. Svcs.	% Racial Min. Clnts. Low <30%	% Racial Min. Clnts. Med. 30-70	% Racial Min. Clnts. High >70%	% Public Asst. Clnts. Low <30%	% Public Asst. Clnts. Med. 30-70	% Public Asst. Clnts. High >70%	Annual Budget Low <$250K	Annual Budget Med.	Annual Budget High >$1M.
Increased governmental controls (n = 71)	28	30	24	42	27	30	6	24	29	32	15	31	35	27	19	33
More adversarial relationships with government agency staff (n = 71)	23	17	32	29	36	15	13	35	14	23	15	17	35	40	31	13*
Increased advocacy for clients (n = 71)	55	57	52	71	55	35	56	47	52	65	46	52	69	47	69	54

^ Significant Chi-square difference (p <= .05)
* Significant linear association (p <= .05)
** Significant linear association (p <= .01)
# Com. = Community/Multi-Service; Adv/Info = Advocacy/Info/Education; MH/SA = Mental Health/Substance Abuse; and Emg. Svcs = Emergency Services

agencies, which hasn't increased substantially during the past four years, whereas welfare reform brought about new relationships and tensions for Washtenaw County organizations.

DISCUSSION

Despite the fact that Michigan's nonprofit organizations have been working in an era of welfare reform since the early 1990s, this study confirmed previous research findings that the 1996 PRWORA has had a substantial impact on the ability of nonprofit organizations to meet the increased expectations and the growing demand for services. Many respondents–regardless of location or service type–frequently expressed concern that their agencies were unable to keep up with increases in client demands–demands that they frequently attributed to the effects of welfare reform. These effects have been particularly pronounced among people of color and those who are homeless, disabled, or in abject poverty. They are also reflected in the large increases in client referrals reported by most agencies, especially for emergency services and longer and/or more frequent contact with clients.

The research also found that nonprofits have made significant changes in the nature and number of their primary program activities in response to welfare reform. Close to half (44%) of the participating organizations reported changes in program objectives and one-third indicated changes in program outcomes due to welfare reform. These changes were particularly striking in those agencies that focused on meeting emergency needs and that served high proportions of TANF recipients. One respondent remarked, "[w]e have had a 30-40% increase in the homeless population and similar increases for survival services. Staff works many unpaid hours. This system is inhumane." Many agencies have expanded existing programs and added new ones, which requires staff to adjust to new responsibilities and additional workloads.

In addition, over half of the respondents reported that welfare policy changes had affected the size and nearly half reported an impact on the sources of their agencies' budgets. Although competition has increased, funding appears to be available for service areas congruent with the goals of PRWORA, such as job training and child care, but other needs like emergency services, substance abuse programs, and mental health care are often underfunded. These effects were particularly dramatic among organizations that serve large percentages of racial minority and public assistance clients.

The study also confirmed that welfare reform has altered the relationship between some nonprofits and government agencies, although not to the same extent as reported in earlier research. This difference may be explained by Michigan's adoption of many welfare reform measures prior to the passage of the PRWORA. While most respondents reported increased accountability requirements, only about one-fourth reported an increase in government control or experienced increased adversarial relationships with public welfare staff. Yet, a majority reported the need to engage in more client advocacy. With their direct involvement with low-income populations, nonprofit human service organizations are uniquely situated to advocate for just and realistic social polices, even if that requires, at times, assuming a conflicting relationship with public officials. In this sense, the value of nonprofits extends beyond their traditional service provision role to that of coordinator of resources, both human and material, which can influence the public debate surrounding poverty.

IMPLICATIONS AND CONCLUSIONS

The research findings point to some serious concerns regarding the future of nonprofit service provision in the United States and the low-income populations they serve, but they also highlight the role of nonprofit organizations as potentially powerful social advocates. Currently, the nonprofits that are most likely to address the most severe economic and social consequences of welfare reform–those that primarily serve racial minority and public assistance clients, whether in urban or non-urban settings–are increasingly unable, despite their best efforts, to respond adequately to the serious challenges they face. In the changing social service environment, small agencies and those that respond to clients' emergency needs are particularly vulnerable. Unlike their larger and more mainstream counterparts, they have less access to critical information, less flexibility in developing alternative staffing patterns, and fewer options to generate new resources.

Contrary to the general perception that declining welfare rolls are an indication that PRWORA has successfully addressed economic hardships, our research reveals that many of these individuals and families continue to struggle and increasingly rely on nonprofit organizations for assistance. In response, numerous respondents spoke of the need to develop new definitions of "success" that move beyond a decline in the welfare rolls, such as examining the consequences of policy changes on children and families. One executive commented, "The state brags about reducing the number of people on public assistance but they [sic] are not measuring an increase in the homeless population." Others were even more pessimistic about the future. According to one respondent, "We should be trying to eliminate poverty and not the poor, which is what welfare reform is slowly doing." These comments reflect respondents' frustration with PRWORA's incentive structure that rewarded states for achieving reductions in their public welfare roles, with no regard for the economic disposition of the former recipient. Switching the emphasis towards poverty and hardship reduction would represent a fundamental shift in current welfare policy and a major victory for those involved in the fight against poverty. To this end, nonprofit organizations constitute a tremendous actual and potential asset for advocacy through the mass mobilization of their clients, staff, donors, and the countless members of the communities in which they serve. Additionally, the existing inter-organizational service and information collaboratives facilitate their capacity for effective collective action. As PRWORA enters reauthorization, nonprofit social service organizations must bring an informed and concentrated force to bear on the discourse.

Additionally, some participants expressed frustration during the focus groups over the state's failure to use all of its federal funds to provide services for current or former TANF recipients while their organizations struggled to make ends meet and satisfy the increased needs of clients. Respondents were aware that Michigan and many other states had not spent substantial portions of the TANF block grants (Lazere, 2000, Stahl, 2000; DeParle, 1999). This practice represents a short-term resource allocation problem and weakens the argument for maintaining substantial social service funding when TANF is reauthorized in 2002. While organizations reported engaging in increased advocacy on behalf of their clients, there may also be a need for greater advocacy on behalf of the nonprofit organizations themselves to ensure that they receive the necessary funding if they are expected to "pick up" where the public social safety net has left off.

Finally, lobbying for continued or increased funding will not fully address some of the primary concerns expressed throughout our research project. Although many organizations reported substantial increases in the size of their budgets, there is once again a growing recognition that the private sector cannot replace the public sector as the nation's primary social safety net. The public policy debate needs to include a greater discussion of the capacity of nonprofit organizations to take on this enhanced role in the social safety net as well as the potential social and administrative costs of such an arrangement. Previous research has raised concerns regarding some of these costs such as a reduction in the nonprofit sector's ability to engage in substantial advocacy work (Young, 1999; Ryan, 1999; Smith and Lipsky, 1993) and promote civil society virtues (Alexander, Nank, and Stivers, 1999).

While our research cannot definitively evaluate these core issues, the findings from our study offer evidence of a strained social safety net and providers that are very apprehensive of the future. Respondents' comments revealed widespread acknowledgment that even though the U.S. experienced the "best of all possible worlds" during the recent economic boom, demand still outstripped the capacity of a number of organizations, especially for emergency service organizations. While we have not experienced widespread rioting in the streets as some predicted when the PRWORA was passed, clearly we need to provide further support for the nation's nonprofit human service organizations and realistically assess their appropriate role in the social safety net of the 21st century as they attempt to address the needs of the "other America."

NOTES

1. It is also important to note that the survey data were collected during the spring and summer of 2000–prior to the recent economic recession and the post-September 11th increase in national security concerns. The social service providers we interviewed, however, recognized that the "good times" of the 1990s would come to an end at some point. This concerned them deeply since many organizations were already facing increased demands for services, especially emergency services, even while unemployment levels were at historic lows.

With the slowing of the national economy, Michigan's seasonally adjusted unemployment rate increased almost 2% (3.8 to 5.7) between November 2000 and November 2001 (U.S. Department of Labor, 2001). Along with this rising unemployment, Michigan's welfare caseloads have increased 5.9% between June and November of 2001 (Family Independence Agency, 2001). Economic difficulties have also prompted a growing need for a variety of emergency services. The recently released report from the U.S. Conference of Mayors noted a sharp increase in the requests for emergency food assistance and shelter throughout the nation (an average increase of 23% and 13% respectively; U.S. Conference of Mayors, 2001). All participating cities expected requests for assistance to increase during 2002.

Therefore, the pressures facing the nonprofit sector organizations have quite probably increased during the period of time since the survey data was originally collected. Additionally, there is some concern that the outpouring of generosity following the September 11 attacks may have diverted funds away from the local nonprofit organizations that must address the economic and physical hardships within many communities.

2. Five child-care/preschool organizations were removed from the overall analysis since all of these organizations were located in Washtenaw County and as a whole, they did not serve low-income populations and had minimal connection to changes in welfare policy. This reduced the survey sample size to 77 organizations, 30 from Washtenaw and 47 from Wayne County.

REFERENCES

Abramovitz, M. (2002, in press). *In jeopardy: The impact of welfare reform on nonprofit human service agencies in New York City*, New York: United Way.

Abramovitz, M. (2000). *Under attack, fighting back: Women and welfare in the United States*, New York: Monthly Review Press.

Albelda, R. (1996). Farewell to welfare: But not to poverty, *Dollars and Sense 208*, 16-19.

Alexander, J. (1999). The impact of devolution on nonprofits: A multiphase study of social service organizations, *Nonprofit Management and Leadership 10 (1)4*, 57-70.

Alexander, J., Nank, R., and Stivers, C. (1999). Implications of welfare reform: Do nonprofit survival strategies threaten civil society? *Nonprofit and Voluntary Sector Quarterly 26 (4)*, 452-475.

Allen, K. and Kirby, M. (2000). *Unfinished business: Why cities matter to welfare reform*, Washington, DC: The Brookings Institute.

Besharov, D.J., Germanis, P., and Rossi, P.H. (1997). *Evaluating welfare reform: A guide for scholars and practitioners*, College Park, MD: University of Maryland.

Bischoff, U. (2001). *The impact of welfare reform on inter-organizational relationships among nonprofit organizations*, unpublished doctoral dissertation, Philadelphia: University of Pennsylvania.

Bloom, D. (1997). *After AFDC: Welfare-to-work choices and challenges for states*, New York: Manpower Demonstration Research Corporation.

Briggs, R. (1999, February 8). Civic, church leaders map plans for welfare changes, *The Philadelphia Inquirer*, B1-2.

Burt, M., Pindus, N., and Capizzano, J. (2000). *The social safety net at the beginning of federal welfare reform: Organization of and access to social services for low-income families*, Washington, DC: The Urban Institute.

Carnochan, S. and Austin, M. (1999, September). *Implementing welfare reform and guiding organizational change*, Berkeley, CA: Bay Area Social Services Consortium.

Cnaan, R., Boddie, S. and Wineburg, R. (1999). *The newer deal: Social work and religion in partnership*, New York: Columbia University Press.

DeParle, J. (1999, August 28). *States struggle to use windfall born of shifts in welfare law*, New York: New York Times, A1, A20.

DiPadova, L. (2000). *Utah's charitable organizations face welfare reform: Concerns of charitable leaders*, Salt Lake City: Center for Public Policy and Administration.

Eisenger, P. (1999). Food pantries and welfare reform: Estimating the effect. *Focus 20(3)*, 23-28.

Family Independence Agency (2000). *Assistance payments statistics*. Lansing, MI.

Family Independence Agency. (2001). *Monthly Trend of Key Statistics: September 2001*. Lansing, MI.

Fink, B. and Widom, R. (2001). *Social Service Organizations and Welfare Reform*. New York: Manpower Demonstration Research Corporation.

Jencks, C. (1996). Can we replace welfare with work? in Darby, M., ed., *Reducing poverty in America: Views and approaches*, Thousand Oaks, CA: Sage Publiations, 69-81.

Johnson, A.K. (1998). The revitalization of community practice: Characteristics, competencies, and curricula for community-based services, *Journal of Community Practice 5(3)*, 37-62.

Kittay, E.F. (1998). Dependency, equality, and welfare, *Feminist studies 24(1)*, 32-43.

Lazere, E. (2000). *Welfare balances after three years of TANF block grants: Unspent TANF funds at the end of federal fiscal year 1999*, Washington, DC: Center on Budget and Policy Priorities.

Meyer, D.R. and Cancian, M. (1998). Economic well-being following an exit from aid to families with dependent children, *Journal of Marriage and the Family 60(2)*, 479-492.

Michigan League for Human Services (1998). *Report on welfare reform in Michigan*, Lansing: Michigan League.

Perlmutter, F. (1997). *From welfare to work: Corporate initiatives and welfare reform*, New York: Oxford University Press.

Raffel, J. (1998). *TANF, Act 35, and Pennsylvania's new welfare system*, Philadelphia: 21st Century League.

Riccio, J. and Orenstein, A. (1996). Understanding best practices for operating welfare-to-work programs, *Evaluation Review 20 (1)*, 3-28.

Ryan, W. P. (1999). The new landscape for nonprofits. *Harvard Business Review, 77(1)*, 127-136.

Seefeldt, K., Pavetti, L., Maguire K., and Kirby G. (1998). *Income support and social services for low-income people in Michigan*, Washington, DC: The Urban Institute.

Smith, S. R. and Lipsky, M. (1993). *Nonprofits for Hire*. Cambridge, MA: Harvard University Press.

Stahl, L. (2000). $175 million to help poor goes unspent: State defends its reserve of federal welfare funds, *The Dallas Morning News*, March 13.

Swigonski, M.E. (1996). Women, poverty and welfare reform: A challenge to social workers, *Affilia 11(1)*, 95-110.

U.S. Bureau of the Census (1990, 1995, 1998, 1999, 2000). *Population statistics*, Washington, DC: U.S. Government Printing Office.

U.S. Bureau of the Census (1997). *Small Area Income and Poverty Estimate*, Washington, DC: U.S. Government Printing Office.

U.S. Conference of Mayors. (2001). *A Status Report on Hunger and Homelessness in America's Cities: 2001*. Washington, DC: Author.

U.S. Department of Health and Human Services (2000). *Change in TANF caseloads*. Washington, DC: Administration for Children & Families.

U.S. Department of Health and Human Services (2000). *Characteristics and financial circumstances of TANF recipients: Fiscal year 1999*, Washington, DC: Administration of Children and Families.

U.S. Department of Labor. (2001). *Regional and State Employment and Unemployment: November 2001*. Washington, DC: Bureau of Labor Statistics.

U.S. Senate. (1996). *Filling the gap: Can private institutions do it?* Vol. 96-S541-18. Senate Committee on Labor and Human Resources.

Withorn, A. and Jons, P. (1999). *Worrying about Welfare Reform.* Boston: Boston Area Academics Working Group on Poverty.

Young, D. (1999). Complementary, supplementary, or adversarial? A theoretical and historical examination of nonprofit-government relations in the United States, in Boris, E. and Steuerle, E., eds., *Nonprofits and government: Collaboration and conflict*, Washington, DC: Urban Institute Press, 31-67.

Gender Differences in the Economic Well-Being of Nonaged Adults in the United States

Martha N. Ozawa
Hong-Sik Yoon

SUMMARY. The attainment of economic parity between men and women has been a focal point of the women's movements in many countries. How much worse off are women economically? What are the net, gender differences in economic well-being when other factors are taken into account? What factors explain the level of economic well-being of women compared to men's? This article reports the results of a study of the gender differences in the economic well-being of women and men in the United States from 1969 to 1999. The major findings are that the gender differential in economic well-being widened during these decades; women's economic well-being was more adversely affected by non-married status than men's; the increasing educational attainment of women offset the adverse effect of marital dissolution on them; and women continued to pay a higher price for caring for children than did men. Implications for policy are discussed. *[Article copies available for a fee from The Haworth Document Delivery Service: 1-800-HAWORTH. E-mail address: <docdelivery@haworthpress.com> Website: <http://www.HaworthPress.com> © 2003 by The Haworth Press, Inc. All rights reserved.]*

Martha N. Ozawa, PhD, is Bettie Bofinger Brown Professor of Social Policy, George Warren Brown School of Social Work, Washington University, St. Louis, MO 63130-4899.

Hong-Sik Yoon is a PhD candidate, George Warren Brown School of Social Work, Washington University, St. Louis, MO 63130-4899.

[Haworth co-indexing entry note]: "Gender Differences in the Economic Well-Being of Nonaged Adults in the United States." Ozawa, Martha N., and Hong-Sik Yoon. Co-published simultaneously in *Journal of Poverty* (The Haworth Press, Inc.) Vol. 7, No. 1/2, 2003, pp. 97-122; and: *Rediscovering the Other America: The Continuing Crisis of Poverty and Inequality in the United States* (ed: Keith M. Kilty, and Elizabeth A. Segal) The Haworth Press, Inc., 2003, pp. 97-122. Single or multiple copies of this article are available for a fee from The Haworth Document Delivery Service [1-800-HAWORTH, 9:00 a.m. - 5:00 p.m. (EST). E-mail address: docdelivery@haworthpress.com].

KEYWORDS. Gender differences, economic well-being, education, marital status, children

The goal of the War on Poverty, initiated by President Lyndon Johnson in the 1960s, was to reduce poverty among the American people. The subsequent decades, as prophesied by Gans (1973), saw the beginning of the public quest for more economic equality between men and women and between minority and majority groups. Since then, women's movements to achieve greater economic and social equality have spread all over the world, and the Fourth World Conference on Women, held in Beijing in 1995, called for action to achieve greater equality. This commitment was reaffirmed at the "Beijing +5" special session of the United Nations General Assembly in 2000.

With this as a backdrop, we ask: How are American women and men living economically? What are the gender differences in economic well-being in the United States?

This article reports differences in the economic well-being of women and men in the United States from 1969 to 1999. In particular, it describes the findings of our study on the following specific questions:

1. What were the differences in the economic well-being of women and men in 1969, 1979, 1989, and 1999?
2. What was the degree of economic inequality among women and men in 1969, 1979, 1989, and 1999?
3. What was the net difference in the economic well-being of women and men in 1969, 1979, 1989, and 1999, when age, race-ethnicity, marital status, number of children, and education were held constant?
4. How did age, race-ethnicity, marital status, number of children, and education correlate with the economic well-being of women and men?

BACKGROUND

The economic well-being of American women is determined by multiple forces. Among them are women's earnings, marital status, number of children and the impact of public income transfers.

Increasing earnings of women. With the advent of a service-oriented and high-technology economy, which characterized the post-World War II U.S. economy, the rate of labor force participation among women increased greatly (Smith, 1989; Smith & Ward, 1989). From 1970 to 1999, the participation rate of women increased 39 percent, from 43.3 percent to 60.0 percent, while that of men decreased 6 percent, from 79.7 percent to 74.7 percent (U.S. Bureau of the Census, 2000b, Table 645, p. 404). Furthermore, the increase in the participation rate of married women with children was even greater–77 percent–from 39.7 percent to 70.1 percent (U.S. Bureau of the Census, 2000b, Table 653, p. 409).

As more and more women entered the labor market, their levels of earnings increased as well. The median earnings per week of full-time female workers increased 10.3 percent, from $429 in 1985 to $473 in 1999 (in 1999 dollars). In contrast, the median earnings per week of full-time male workers decreased 1.6 percent, from $629 in 1985 to $618 in 1999 (in 1999 dollars). Even among highly paid workers, the gender differential narrowed. For example, Wood, Corcoran, and Courant (1993) found that 15 years after graduation from law school, the gender differential in annual earnings was 13 percent when law school performance, marital and fertility history, experience, and job setting (business versus government, size of firms, and so on) were controlled.

The relatively favorable development in women's earning power over the years has been affected by women's increasing educational attainment. In 1970, only 8.1 percent of women had four or more years of college, compared with 13.5 percent of men. But in 1999, 23.1 percent of women versus 27.5 percent of men attained this level of education. Moreover, in 1999 the educational attainment of black and Hispanic women was higher than that of their male counterparts. That is, 16.4 percent of black women, compared with 14.2 percent of black men, and 11.0 percent of Hispanic women, compared with 10.7 percent of Hispanic men, had attained this level of education (U.S. Bureau of Census, 2000b, Table 250, p. 157).

Marital status. Differential marital statuses affect the economic well-being of women more strongly than that of men. Divorce, in particular, affects women adversely. Duncan and Hoffman (1991) found that family income (measured by the income-to-needs ratio) fell 25 percent for divorced women but only 3 percent for divorced men. Ozawa and Hong (2000) showed that the income status (measured by the income-to-needs ratio) of nonaged women declined 32 percent as a result of divorce. The adverse impact of divorce is reflected in the disproportionally low levels of economic well-being of female-headed households, and their relative economic disadvantage has persisted for the past two decades. In both 1980 and 1999, the income of female-headed households was only 46 percent of the income of married-couple households (U.S. Bureau of the Census, 2001).

The economic disadvantage of households headed by divorced women is compounded by the inefficient collection of child support payments from noncustodial fathers. In 1995, of all custodial mothers who were awarded child support payments, only 69 percent received them, and 31 percent received none. Among those who received such payments, 57 percent received full payments, and 53 percent received partial payments. In that year, child support payments ($3,767) constituted only 17 percent of the total money income ($21,829) of female-headed families (U.S. Bureau of the Census, 2000b, Table 631, p. 394).

Effect of children. While more and more women with children are participating in the labor market, children affect the economic well-being of women adversely. Other things being equal, women–married or nonmarried–pay a price for having children. Hill (1988) found that during the 1984-86 period, having children decreased the work time of married women by 425 hours a year and that of unmarried women by 244 hours a year. In contrast, the existence of children has no statistically significant impact on male labor supply (Triest 1990). Furthermore, a study by McNeil, Lamas, and Haber (1987) showed that the hourly wages of women with children were significantly lower than those of childless women with similar educational backgrounds. Looking at the effect of children on women's lifetime earnings, Ozawa and Wang (1993) found that controlling for education, the amount of lifetime earnings of white women decreased significantly and persistently as the number of children increased from zero to 1, to 2, to 3, to 4 or more. The lifetime earnings of black women, however, were affected adversely only when the women had 4 or more children.

Children affect women's economic well-being in another way. Because children cause household expenditures to increase, the economic well-being (measured by the income-to-needs ratio) of women declines. These two adverse effects–lower earnings and larger household expenditures–are acutely felt particularly by female heads of households, who must live on one paycheck and have greater expenditures.

Public income transfers. There is evidence that the U.S. system of public income transfers–both the social security system and Temporary Assistance for Needy Families (TANF, formerly Aid to Families with Dependent Children [AFDC])–is increasingly eluding the lives of women with children who head their households. With regard to the social security program, over the years, the probability of female-headed families with children being covered by Survivors Insurance declined as more families became female headed not because of the death of their breadwinners, but because of separation, divorce, or nonmarriage (Social

Security Administration, 2000 Table 6.A1, p. 233). With regard to welfare, Moffitt (1992) noted that the real value of AFDC benefits rose steadily from 1960 to 1975, leveled off, and then fell in the late 1970s and early 1980s, leveling off again in the mid-1980s. A study by the Congressional Research Service (Solomon, 1992) found that in constant 1992 dollars, the median state's maximum AFDC payment for a family of four declined from $796 in 1979 to $435 in 1992, a reduction of 45.4 percent. There is no reason to expect that the TANF payment level has increased commensurate with inflation because the federal government allows states to maintain TANF payments at the previous AFDC payment levels.

As we described, women's economic well-being depends on multiple factors. Some factors make women's economic well-being higher, and some do not. In particular, women's increasing labor force participation and earnings have positive effects on women's economic well-being, whereas divorce and nonmarriage have negative effects. In addition, women pay an economic price for having children more than do men. Furthermore, there are indications that the U.S. system of public income transfers is becoming less effective in improving women's economic well-being. Although this information is informative, it does not help us discern the *net* difference in the economic well-being of women and men. The study reported in this article estimated the net differential in the economic well-being of women and men, taking into account age, race-ethnicity, marital status, the number of children, and education.

METHODOLOGY

Source of Data

The data used in this study came from the 1970, 1980, 1990, and 2000 Current Population Surveys (CPSs) of the civilian noninstitutional population. The four surveys interviewed the following number of people aged 14 and over: 1970 survey, 104,400 people; 1980 survey, 135,000 people; 1990 survey, 114,500 people; and 2000 survey, 133,700 people. The CPS collects data on each respondent's level and sources of income, demographic background, education, living arrangements, employment, unemployment, wages and hours of work, occupation, industry in which employed, participation in publicly supported programs, and number of children in the family. The data are organized to enable researchers to investigate the economic lives of the U.S. population on the basis of individuals, families, or households. Because data for income are always for the year preceding the survey year, the variable economic well-being we developed is based on the income data for one year previous to the year of the survey. All non-income-related variables are for the year of survey (U.S. Bureau of the Census, 1984a, 1984b, 1991, 2000a). For our study, we selected women and men aged 18 through 64.

Conceptual Framework for Economic Well-Being

In our study, economic well-being was measured by the income-to-needs ratio, which was operationalized as the ratio of family income to poverty-line income. For example, an income-to-needs ratio of 2 means that the respondents were living at twice the poverty-line income. This procedure assumed that all the people in the same family had the same economic well-being. Thus, if the respondent was married, both spouses were assumed to have the same economic well-being. One advantage of using the income-to-needs ratio instead of other indicators, such as per capita family income, is that it incorporates economies of scale as well as family size, making it possible to compare more precisely the economic well-being of one person with that of another person, regardless of the size of the families from which both came. Another advantage is that the income-to-needs ratio implicitly deals with price fluctuations, so it is possible to compare economic well-being in various years.

Definitions of Variables

Dependent variable. The dependent variable for this study was the economic well-being of nonaged adults aged 18 to 64. As we stated earlier, this variable was measured by the income-to-needs ratio, which was obtained by dividing family income by poverty-line income.

Independent variable. The major independent variable was gender. A dummy variable was developed for this variable, assigning the value of 1 to women and zero to men.

Independent variables used as controls. To net out the effect of gender on the economic well-being of nonaged adults, we included the following variables as controls: age, race-ethnicity, marital status, number of children, and education. Age and number of children were continuous variables and are self-explanatory. To measure race-ethnicity, we developed two dummy variables–one for the black respondents and the other for the Hispanic respondents–assigning the white respondents to the reference group. Because of the lack of information on Hispanic versus non-Hispanic ethnic status in the 1970 CPS, we dichotomized race into white versus nonwhite in that year. To measure marital status, we developed three dummy variables for divorced-separated, widowed, and never-married respondents, assigning married respondents to the reference group. To measure the level of education, we developed three dummy variables for those with less than a high school education, those with some college education, and those with a college education, assigning those with a high school education to the reference group.

Analysis and Presentation of Data

First, we generated descriptive statistics on the backgrounds of the respondents from each survey. Second, we generated descriptive statistics on the income-to-needs ratios for 1969, 1979, 1989, and 1999 and calculated the percentage changes in the ratios from 1969 to 1979, from 1979 to 1989, from 1989 to 1999, and from 1969 to 1999. Third, we generated descriptive statistics on income inequality (measured by Gini coefficients) for 1969, 1979, 1989, and 1999 and observed the percentage changes between these years. The Gini coefficient ranges from zero to 1; the higher the Gini coefficient, the greater the inequality (see Plotnick, 1995). We used the weight variable that was developed by the Bureau of the Census to generate descriptive statistics on all variables. This procedure was needed to adjust for the sampling, poststratification, and nonresponse biases in the CPS data sets.

Fourth, we conducted a series of ordinary least square (OLS) regression analyses on the economic well-being of women and men. To net out the effect of gender, we included, as controls, age, race-ethnicity, marital status, number of children, and education. We further conducted OLS regression analyses for women and men separately. This statistical procedure was used to investigate how age, race-ethnicity, marital status, number of children, and education were related to women's and men's economic well-being. For conducting OLS regression analyses, we transformed income-to-needs ratios into natural logs because the distribution of income-to-needs ratios was skewed.

FINDINGS

Descriptive Statistics

Backgrounds of the respondents. Three trends emerged from Table 1. First, the level of women's education increased faster than the men's over the decades. Thus, in 2000, the percentage of women who had at least some college education (55.3 percent) surpassed that of men (54.6 percent).

Second, the marital statuses of women and men differed considerably. Women were more likely to be divorced-separated or widowed in all the years under investigation, men were more likely to be never married than women in all these years, and men were more likely to be married in 1970 and 1980, but in 1990 and 2000, both groups are almost equally married. It was noteworthy that although the percentage of women who were divorced-separated was consistently higher than that of men, the rate of growth in this marital status was much higher for men: From 1970 to 2000, the proportion of men who were divorced increased 588 percent, compared with 159 percent among women. The reverse was true with regard to the rate of growth in the never-married status: Although the percentage of women who were never married was consistently lower than that of men, the rate of growth in this marital status from 1970 to 2000 was slightly higher among women (169 percent) than among men (157 percent).

Third, the population of nonaged adults became more diverse over the years. Looking at the female population, 89.1 percent were white in 1970, but 74.4 percent were white in 2000. The growth of Hispanic nonaged adults was enormous. Whereas only 5.6 percent of the female population were Hispanic in 1980, 11.8 percent were Hispanic in 2000–a 111 percent increase. This phenomenal increase in the proportion of Hispanic people was due to high rates of immigration and fertility (see Ozawa, 1997).

Level of economic well-being (income-to-needs ratios). As Table 2 indicates, the level of women's economic well-being, which was measured by income-to-needs ratios, was persistently lower than the men's in the years under investigation. The differential was 2.6 percent, 8.8 percent, 10.0 percent, and 8.7 percent, respectively, in 1969, 1979, 1989, and 1999. Furthermore, the rate of increase in women's income-to-needs ratio from one decade to the other was smaller, except for the decade 1989 to 1999. All told, the rate of increase in women's income-to-needs ratio from 1969 to 1999 was 27.1 percent, compared with a 35.6 percent for men's.

Income inequality. Income inequality was measured by the Gini coefficient, as stated earlier. Table 3 shows that the degree of income inequality among women was higher than that among men by 7.0 percent, 7.5 percent, 8.5 percent, and 6.1 percent, respectively, in 1969, 1979, 1989, and 1999. Furthermore, the rate of growth in in-

TABLE 1. Backgrounds of the Respondents (percentage)

	1970 Female (n = 35,852)	1970 Male (n = 32,551)	1980 Female (n = 52,585)	1980 Male (n = 48,495)	1990 Female (n = 46,852)	1990 Male (n = 43,473)	2000 Female (n = 39,427)	2000 Male (n = 37,189)
Age (year)								
20 to 29	27.6	25.6	31.1	32.0	26.8	27.3	22.7	23.1
30 to 39	23.0	22.5	24.3	24.9	28.6	29.3	25.8	26.2
40 to 49	23.8	24.1	18.8	17.9	21.5	21.5	26.2	26.2
50 to 64	25.7	27.8	26.8	25.3	23.1	21.9	25.4	24.5
Race								
White	89.1	90.8	82.7	84.4	76.2	77.7	74.4	76.0
Black (nonwhite)[a]	10.9	9.2	11.7	10.1	15.8	14.0	13.8	11.7
Hispanic			5.6	5.5	8.0	8.4	11.8	12.3
Marital status								
Married	82.4	87.1	67.5	68.9	62.9	62.9	60.4	60.2
Widowed	3.8	0.6	5.3	1.0	4.2	0.8	3.1	0.8
Divorced-separated	5.8	1.7	11.9	8.0	14.3	10.2	15.0	11.7
Never married	8.0	10.6	15.3	22.1	18.6	26.0	21.5	27.3

105

TABLE 1 (continued)

	1970 Female (n = 35,852)	1970 Male (n = 32,551)	1980 Female (n = 52,585)	1980 Male (n = 48,495)	1990 Female (n = 46,852)	1990 Male (n = 43,473)	2000 Female (n = 39,427)	2000 Male (n = 37,189)
Number of children								
None	38.8	38.6	49.6	53.7	53.3	59.6	55.2	61.7
One or two	38.7	39.2	39.0	36.0	37.6	32.5	35.8	30.5
Three or more	22.5	22.3	11.5	10.3	9.1	7.9	9.1	7.8
Education								
Less than high school	35.4	36.2	23.6	23.5	16.4	17.3	12.2	13.3
High school	42.2	32.3	41.7	33.1	38.6	34.3	32.5	32.2
Some college	14.3	17.3	20.4	22.8	23.6	21.9	30.1	27.8
College education	8.2	14.2	14.4	20.6	21.4	26.5	25.2	26.8

Note: [a]The "nonwhite" category is only for 1969.

TABLE 2. Mean Income-to-Needs Ratio, 1969 to 1999

	1969	1979	1989	1999
	\multicolumn{4}{c}{Income-to-Needs Ratio}
All	3.38	3.69	3.99	4.51
Women	3.39	3.54	3.79	4.31
Men	3.48	3.88	4.21	4.72

	1969 to 1979	1979 to 1989	1989 to 1999	1969 to 1999
	\multicolumn{4}{c}{Percentage Change}
All	9.2	8.1	13.0	33.4
Women	4.4	7.1	13.7	27.1
Men	11.5	8.5	12.1	35.6

equality among women was larger from 1969 to 1979 and from 1979 to 1989, but considerably smaller from 1989 to 1999, compared with the rate of growth among men. All told, from 1969 to 1999, the Gini coefficient increased 23.6 percent among women, but 24.7 percent among men.

OLS Multiple Regression Analysis

Before we present the results of the OLS multiple regression analyses, it is important to recognize that regression coefficients in such analyses, in which the dependent variable is transformed into a natural log and independent variables take the form of dummy variables, need to be transformed. Halvorsen and Palmquiest (1980) argued that in such a situation, one could not use the regression coefficients to evaluate the relative effect of the independent variable on the dependent variable; rather, one would need to use transformed coefficients. In econometric terms, they argued:

$C = ln(1 + g)$
$e^c = 1 + g$
therefore,
$g = e^c - 1$
where C = regression coefficent and g = relative effect.

TABLE 3. Gini Coefficient of the Income-to-Needs Ratio, 1969 to 1999

	1969	1979	1989	1999
	\multicolumn{4}{c}{Gini Coefficient}
All	0.340	0.350	0.395	0.422
Women	0.351	0.359	0.410	0.434
Men	0.328	0.334	0.378	0.409
	\multicolumn{4}{c}{Percentage Change}
	1969 to 1979	1979 to 1989	1989 to 1999	1969 to 1999
All	2.9	12.9	6.8	24.1
Women	2.3	14.2	5.9	23.6
Men	1.8	13.2	8.2	24.7

Following this equation and applying the coefficient of 0.363, for example, one finds the relative effect g to be 0.438, which can be interpreted as 43.8 percent greater. Thus, in the data analysis that follows, we used the procedure specified by Halvorsen and Palmquiest. We calculated the values of the relative effect g (expressed in percentage by multiplying the transformed coefficient by 100) for all coefficients for dummy variables in the OLS multiple regression analyses that involved the natural log of income-to-needs ratios as the dependent variable and dummy variables as independent variables. (This transformation was not required for independent variables that were interval.) We listed relative effects after t values.

OLS multiple regression analysis of the income-to-needs ratio (log): All. Table 4 shows the net effect of gender on the economic well-being of nonaged adults in 1969, 1979, 1989, and 1999. It indicates that the gender differential in income-to-needs ratios widened from 3.9 percent in 1969, to 8.6 percent in 1979, and to 15.3 percent in 1989 and slightly declined to 15.0 percent in 1999, to the disadvantage of women.

It is noteworthy that the race-ethnicity differential in income-to-needs ratios was higher than the gender differential in every year under investigation. As of 1999, black persons were still 24.1 percent worse off than white persons. The relative economic disadvantage of never-married persons increased over the years, with the result that their income-to-needs ratio was 48.8 percent lower than that of married persons in 1999, com-

TABLE 4. OLS Multiple Regression Analysis of the Income-to-Needs Ratio (log): All

	1969 Coefficient (t)	1969 Relative Effect (%)	1979 Coefficient (t)	1979 Relative Effect (%)	1989 Coefficient (t)	1989 Relative Effect (%)	1999 Coefficient (t)	1999 Relative Effect (%)
Intercept	0.855***		1.232***		1.109***		1.079***	
Age (year)	0.010*** (30.82)		0.005*** (16.39)		0.008*** (16.43)		0.007*** (12.41)	
Female	−0.040*** (−5.34)	−3.9	−0.091*** (−13.45)	−8.6	−0.166*** (−17.71)	−15.3	−0.162*** (−14.41)	−15.0
Race								
Black-nonwhite[a]	−0.392*** (−31.83)	−34.4	−0.335*** (−27.54)	−28.5	−0.483*** (−30.72)	−38.3	−0.275*** (−13.87)	−24.1
Hispanic			−0.194*** (−15.85)	−17.6	−0.401*** (−26.24)	−33.1	−0.270*** (−16.64)	−23.6
(White)								
Marital status								
Divorced-separated	−0.908*** (−47.09)	−59.7	−0.591*** (−51.19)	−44.6	−0.602*** (−40.52)	−45.2	−0.670*** (−38.79)	−48.8
Widowed	−0.502*** (−20.27)	−39.5	−0.630*** (−31.94)	−46.7	−0.596*** (−19.52)	−44.9	−0.601*** (−14.47)	−45.2
Never married	0.081*** (5.93)	8.4	−0.379*** (−36.99)	−32.2	−0.501*** (−35.68)	−39.4	−0.669*** (−40.37)	−48.8

TABLE 4 (continued)

	1969 Coefficient (t)	1969 Relative Effect (%)	1979 Coefficient (t)	1979 Relative Effect (%)	1989 Coefficient (t)	1989 Relative Effect (%)	1999 Coefficient (t)	1999 Relative Effect (%)
(Married)								
Number of children	−0.114*** (−46.87)		−0.165*** (−56.73)		−0.181*** (−39.46)		−0.156*** (−27.96)	
Education								
Less than high school	−0.332*** (−38.04)	−28.3	−0.426*** (−47.67)	−34.7	−0.607*** (−43.57)	−45.5	−0.602*** (−32.43)	−45.2
(High school)								
Some college	0.133*** (11.96)	14.2	0.123*** (13.66)	13.1	0.261*** (21.07)	29.8	0.292*** (20.31)	33.9
College education	0.383*** (30.63)	46.7	0.297*** (30.68)	34.6	0.525*** (42.37)	69.1	0.658*** (43.96)	93.2
R^2	0.167		0.142		0.157		0.137	
F	1,370.16***		1,524.2***		1,474.6***		1,101.5***	
N	68,403		101,080		87,402		76,616	

*$p < .05$, **$p < .01$, ***$p < .001$.
[a]The "nonwhite" category is only for 1969.
Note: t values in parentheses.

pared with an 8.4 percent *advantage* in 1969. The impact of education on the income-to-needs ratio increased considerably over the years. For instance, those with college education had income-to-needs ratios that were 93.2 percent higher than those with a high school education in 1999, compared with a 46.7 percent advantage in 1969. The economic disadvantage of having children became considerably greater from 1969 to 1979 to 1989 and leveled off in 1999. The impact of age was positive in each year under investigation, but over the decades, the degree of the impact declined.

OLS multiple regression analysis of the income-to-needs ratio (log): Comparison between women and men. Tables 5 and 6 show how the independent variables correlate differentially with the income-to-needs ratios of women and men.

Tables 5 and 6 show two important, differential results: the effects of marital status and education. First, with regard to the impact of marital status on economic well-being, although the economic price that women paid for getting divorced, never marrying, or becoming widowed was consistently higher than the price that men paid in every year under investigation, the *trend* in the degree of economic disadvantage associated with divorce/separation and widowhood was in favor of women. For example, the economic disadvantage of divorced-separated women (that is, the relative difference in income-to-needs ratios of divorced-separated women and married women–see Table 5) relative to the disadvantage of divorced-separated men decreased from 7.1 times, to 2.3 times, to 1.7 times, and to 1.6 times in 1967, 1979, 1989, and 1999, respectively (see Table 6). Likewise, the economic disadvantage of widows relative to that of widowers decreased from 2.2 times in 1969, to 1.6 times in 1979, and to 1.1 times in 1989 and leveled off to 1.3 times in 1999.

However, the relative economic disadvantage of never-married women followed an opposite trend. The impact of the never-married status was positive in 1969 on both men and women, but it became negative in 1979 on both men and women and thereafter became increasingly more negative for women than for men, with the result that women's relative economic disadvantage associated with the never-married status was 1.5 times that of men in 1999.

Second, with regard to education, the impact of education was greater on women's income-to-needs ratio in every year under investigation. For example, a college education gave a 52.3 percent, 40.4 percent, 85.5 percent, and 110.4 percent economic advantage to women over those with a high school education in 1969, 1979, 1989, and 1999, respectively. The comparable figures for men were 45.1 percent, 32

TABLE 5. OLS Multiple Regression Analysis of the Income-to-Needs Ratio (log): Women

	1969 Coefficient (t)	1969 Relative Effect (%)	1979 Coefficient (t)	1979 Relative Effect (%)	1989 Coefficient (t)	1989 Relative Effect (%)	1999 Coefficient (t)	1999 Relative Effect (%)
Intercept	0.812***		1.146***		0.878***		0.776***	
Age (year)	0.011*** (20.83)		0.006*** (12.44)		0.010*** (13.75)		0.011*** (13.51)	
Race								
Black-nonwhite[a]	−0.405*** (−21.90)	−33.3	−0.331*** (−19.06)	−28.2	−0.459*** (−21.99)	−36.7	−0.274*** (−9.83)	−24.0
Hispanic			−0.196*** (−10.84)	−17.7	−0.421*** (−18.20)	−34.4	−0.298*** (−12.60)	−25.8
(White)								
Marital status								
Divorced-separated	−1.125** (−46.01)	−67.5	−0.786*** (−50.10)	−54.4	−0.755*** (−36.23)	−53.0	−0.838*** (−35.46)	−56.7
Widowed	−0.558*** (−18.55)	−42.7	−0.698*** (−30.01)	−50.2	−0.620*** (−16.91)	−46.2	−0.697*** (−14.38)	−50.2
Never married	0.004 (0.18)	0.4	−0.478*** (−30.30)	−38.0	−0.625*** (−29.03)	−46.5	−0.850*** (−35.05)	−57.2

(Married)							
Number of children	−0.109*** (−28.55)		−0.159*** (−36.96)		−0.165*** (−24.19)		−0.145*** (−18.23)
Education							
Less than high school	−0.358*** (−27.16)	−30.1	−0.461*** (−35.57)	−36.9	−0.689*** (−32.74)	−49.7	−0.670*** (−24.48)	−48.8
(High school)							
Some college	0.154*** (8.84)	16.6	0.167*** (12.51)	18.1	0.318*** (17.78)	37.3	0.367*** (17.73)	44.3
College education	0.420*** (19.60)	52.3	0.339*** (22.38)	40.4	0.618*** (32.29)	85.5	0.745*** (33.90)	110.4
R^2	0.176		0.163		0.160		0.163
F	850.7***		1,021.9***		889.0***		769.6***
N	35,852		52,584		46,852		39,426

*$p < .05$, **$p < .01$, ***$p < .001$.
[a]The "nonwhite" category is only for 1969.
Note: *t* values in parentheses.

TABLE 6. OLS Multiple Regression Analysis of the Income-to-Needs Ratio (log): Men

	1969 Coefficient (t)	1969 Relative Effect (%)	1979 Coefficient (t)	1979 Relative Effect (%)	1989 Coefficient (t)	1989 Relative Effect (%)	1999 Coefficient (t)	1999 Relative Effect (%)
Intercept	0.826***		1.173***		1.049***		1.117***	
Age (year)	0.010*** (24.99)		0.005*** (12.50)		0.007*** (12.39)		0.004*** (5.58)	
Race								
Black-nonwhite[a]	−0.365*** (−23.53)	−30.6	−0.320*** (−19.11)	−27.4	−0.453*** (−23.81)	−36.4	−0.238*** (−8.45)	−21.2
Hispanic			−0.182*** (−11.17)	−16.6	−0.375*** (−18.67)	−31.3	−0.239*** (−10.93)	−21.3
(White)								
Marital status								
Divorced-separated	−0.100** (−2.99)	−9.5	−0.274*** (−15.82)	−23.9	−0.374*** (−17.30)	−31.2	−0.445*** (−17.54)	−35.9
Widowed	−0.213*** (−3.77)	−19.2	−0.384*** (−8.41)	−31.9	−0.532*** (−7.63)	−41.3	−0.473*** (−5.23)	−37.7
Never married	0.155*** (9.77)	16.8	−0.274*** (−20.90)	−24.0	−0.366*** (−20.32)	−30.6	−0.484*** (−21.48)	−38.4

(Married)							
Number of children	−0.112*** (−38.06)		−0.154*** (−39.52)		−0.163*** (−26.73)		−0.139*** (−17.73)
Education							
Less than high school	−0.303*** (−27.62)	−26.1	−0.386*** (−31.96)	−32.0	−0.532*** (−29.21)	−41.3	−0.534*** (−21.50)	−41.4
(High school)							
Some college	0.120*** (9.03)	12.8	0.088*** (7.37)	9.1	0.213*** (12.92)	23.7	0.230*** (11.64)	25.9
College education	0.373*** (26.49)	45.1	0.278*** (22.66)	32.0	0.473*** (30.14)	60.3	0.602*** (29.73)	82.6
R^2	0.159		0.113		0.134		0.106	
F	683.6***		618.6***		671.8***		441.9***	
N	32,551		48,494		43,473		37,189	

*$p < .05$, **$p < .01$, ***$p < .001$.
[a]The "nonwhite" category is only for 1969.
Note: *t* values in parentheses.

percent, 60.3 percent, and 82.6 percent in 1969, 1979, 1989, and 1999, respectively. Moreover, the positive impact of some college or a college education increased faster for women than for men. From 1969 to 1999, the positive effects of some college and a college education among women increased by 167 percent and 111 percent, respectively, compared with 102 percent and 83 percent, respectively, among men. It is important, however, to observe the increasingly negative effect of less than a high school education on women. Its negative effect on women's income-to-needs ratio increased from 30.1 percent in 1969 to 48.8 in percent in 1999–or a 62 percent deterioration. Such a negative effect on the men's income-to-needs ratio increased from 26.1 percent in 1969 to 41.4 percent in 1999–or a 59 percent deterioration. These data indicate that the variation in the effect of education increased more among women than among men.

The effects of other variables were also noteworthy. Except in 1969, the degree to which children adversely affected the income-to-needs ratio of women was persistently higher than that of men, and the trend worsened in the ensuing decades.

The effect of race-ethnicity on income-to-needs ratio was always greater among women than among men. The black-white differential improved less slowly among women than among men. Specifically, black women's income-to-needs ratio was 28.2 percent lower than that of white women's in 1979 and 24 percent lower in 1999–an improvement of 15 percent. But a similar calculation for men indicated a 23 percent improvement from 1979 to 1999.

The Hispanic-white differential widened considerably among women than among men. In particular, the income-to-needs ratio of Hispanic women was 17.7 percent lower in 1979, and 25.8 percent lower in 1999–a decrease of 46 percent. The comparable figure for men was 28 percent. That the Hispanic-white differential increased was due, in part, to the growth of Hispanic immigration (see Ozawa, 1997): Hispanic immigrants typically have low-income statuses.

The effects of age on income-to-needs ratios differed. Tables 5 and 6 indicate not only that the age effect was larger for women than for men, but that the effect generally stayed stable for women while it decreased for men. These tables indicate that among women, advancement in age was more clearly associated with the increase in their income-to-needs ratios; for men, advancing age meant much smaller increases in their income-to-needs ratios.

DISCUSSION AND CONCLUSIONS

The major findings from this study are that (1) the net gender difference in income statuses of women and men existed in every year under investigation and (2) the net gender difference increased over the years. As of 1999, the net gender difference was 15.0 percent, compared with 3.9 percent in 1969 (see Table 4). A research agenda for the future is why the net gender difference in income statuses of women and men has increased. Changing employment practices may be one area that warrants further study. With the advent of the globalization of and concomitant greater competition in the economy, new terms of employment have emerged (Barker, 1993; duRivage, 1992). The new terms include part-time work, contract work, temporary work, and contingency work, and these terms of employment increased the fastest in service-oriented industries in which female workers predominate (Barker & Christensen, 1998). Cutting across all these terms of employment is intermittent employment and fewer benefits, such as retirement plans, vacation pay, bonuses, options, and noncash fringe benefits (for example, health care coverage and subsidized child care).

It will be important, therefore, to investigate the trend in the proportion of female workers who are subjected to these emerging terms of employment. If the proportion of female workers in such employment terms increased faster than that of male workers, one would expect that such employment practices might have affected, increasingly adversely, the economic standing of women. Furthermore, the findings from future research on the matter would tell us how limited–and inadequate–the often-used indicators, such as the median earnings per week of full-time workers and the median hourly wage, are in measuring the economic standing of women versus men.

In addition to the major finding just mentioned, this study, on the basis of separate regression analyses for women and men, found that women's economic well-being has been affected by two countervailing forces: increasing education and changing marital status. Higher levels of education contributed more effectively to the rise in women's income-to-needs ratios over the four decades we studied relative to that of men's. On the other hand, marital dissolution and nonmarriage have placed greater negative pressures on women's income-to-needs ratios than on men's. In addition, children have always created greater economic hardship on women than on men. Furthermore, the adverse economic impact of having an additional child increased more for women than for men over the years. All this happened in the decades in which the number of children decreased (see Table 1).

One can expect that the configuration of these three forces–education, marital status, and children–will change. As women's educational level further increases and if the rates of divorce and nonmarriage stabilize, women's economic well-being will improve. However, if both women's educational level and rates of divorce and nonmarriage increase, the economic disadvantage of women may stay as it is now. Or controlling for these two factors and if the number of children further decreases and the collection of child support is enforced more strongly and efficiently, women's economic well-being may improve.

An important question that arises from the configuration of these three forces is this: Will women's higher education always force the rates of divorce and nonmarriage to increase, as in the past? Twenty-five years ago, Becker, Landes, and Michael (1977) developed a theory on the division of labor and argued that marriages based on division of labor maximize the benefit of marriage and, therefore, are most stable. This theory implied that women with higher levels of education and, therefore, high earnings are more likely not to marry and, if they do, are more likely to divorce. However, the recent literature (Hochschild, 1989; Nock, 2001) indicates that new generations of adults are establishing a new model of stable marriages, in which both spouses work and both have similar amounts of earnings. That is, stable marriages in contemporary society no longer require a division of labor as theorized by Becker et al. If the new theory of marriage holds true, women's higher education may become positively related to the likelihood and stability of marriage. Future research on marriage and divorce may provide support for such a prediction.

We need to acknowledge the effect of the methodology we used in defining economic well-being on the outcomes of the study. As we stated earlier, economic well-being was measured by the income-to-needs ratio, which was operationalized by dividing family income by the poverty-line income. We assumed that as long as women are married, their income-to-needs ratio is equal to that of their husbands. Therefore, the level of economic well-being is the same for a wife and a husband in the same family. One may argue that as long as women's financial contributions to the family are smaller than men's, women cannot expect to have the same level of economic well-being as can men. However, the intent of this study was to investigate women's economic well-being, regardless of the sources of family income. On this point, we need to continue investigating what the goal of the women's movement really is with regard to greater economic equality between men and women: to improve the well-being of individuals or that of individuals in the context of families? This issue needs to be addressed in future research on women's economic well-being.

Another point that needs to be discussed is the merit of using the income-to-needs ratio as an indicator of economic well-being. As developed by the U.S. Bureau of the Census, this concept incorporates "economies of scale." That is, the needs of a two-person family are defined as 129 percent–not 200 percent–of the needs of a one-person family (Social Security Administration, 2000, p. 130). Thus, two women with the identical amount of earnings, one of whom is married and the other of whom is not married, have considerably different levels of economic well-being. Suppose that both women have annual earnings of $30,000, and one of them is married to a man with annual earnings of $30,000. Then the income-to-needs ratio of the married woman will be 5.4, whereas the income-to-needs ratio of the nonmarried woman will be 3.5. In this case, the economic well-being of the married woman is 54 percent higher than that of the nonmarried woman. Only when per capita family income is used as an indicator of economic well-being are these women's levels of economic well-being identical. We believe, however, that the income-to-needs ratio is a more appropriate indicator of economic well-being than per capita income. The reason, as mentioned earlier, is that the income-to-needs ratio incorporates the economy of scale, but per capita income (which is obtained by dividing family income by the number of persons in the family) does not.

Can the government do anything to help women improve their economic well-being? An important area of intervention is to subsidize the cost of raising children. As this study showed, children impose financial hardship on women, whether the women are married or nonmarried; such hardship is particularly great for nonmarried women who head households. Policy initiatives could be undertaken on several fronts. First, the enforcement of child support should be strengthened. Second, mechanisms for redistributing income to families with children should be expanded. The recent legislation of the $1,000 tax credit per child (the Economic Growth and Tax Relief Reconciliation Act of 2001, P.L. 107-16) seems to be in the right direction. But it has several limitations–especially in relation to channeling financial resources to low-income families. Instead of this tax credit, a children's allowance program should be explored for its political and economic feasibility (see Ozawa & Hong, undated). Furthermore, policy makers should change "unpaid leave" to "paid leave" under the Family and Medical Leave Act of 1993 (P.L. 103-3).

More important, Congress needs to look into the effects of nontraditional terms of employment on workers–especially female workers–and investigate the possible illegality of the unequal treatment of workers who work under the different terms of employment but in the same companies. If such terms of employment are found illegal, certain aspects of employment practices should be prohibited. Even if they are found legal, policy makers should still find ways with which these workers' lives could be protected by developing public provisions, for instance, for health care coverage and liberalized unemployment insurance.

As this study showed, the investigation of gender differences in economic well-being is complex. The future economic well-being of women will depend on the dynamic play of women's education, marital status, the number of children they raise, and, perhaps, the terms of employment under which they work. The major focus of public policy intervention should be on how to help women meet the cost of childbearing and child rearing, on how to compensate women for the years of work they lose because of childbearing and child rearing, and on how to protect women from discriminatory employment practices.

REFERENCES

Barker, K., & Christensen, K. (1998). Controversy and challenges raised by contingent work arrangements. In *Contingent work: American employment relations in transition* (pp. 1-18). Ithaca, NY: ILR Press.

Barker, K. (1993). Changing assumptions and contingent solutions: The costs and benefits of women working full and part-time. *Sex Roles, 28*, 47-71.

Becker, G. S., Landes, M., & Michael, R. (1977). An economic analysis of marital instability. *Journal of Political Economy, 85*, 1141-1187.

Duncan, G., & Hoffman, S. (1991). Economic consequences of marital instability. In M. David & T. Smeeding (Eds.), *Horizontal equity, uncertainty and well-being* (pp. 427-467). Chicago: University of Chicago Press.

duRivage, V. L. (1992). New policies for the part-time and contingent workforce. In V. L. duRivage (Ed.), *New policies for the part-time and contingent workforce* (pp. 89-122). Armonk, NY: M.E. Sharpe.

Gans, H. J. (1973). *More equality*. New York: Pantheon Books.

Hill, M. (1988). *The employment of mothers and the prevention of poverty* (Survey of Income and Participation, Working Paper No. 8826). Washington, DC: U.S. Bureau of the Census.

Halvorsen, R., & Palmquiest, R. (1980). The interpretation of dummy variables in semilogarithmic equations. *American Economic Review, 70*, 474-475.

Hochschild, A. (1989). *The second shift*. New York: Avon Books.

McNeil, J., Lamas, E., & Haber, S. (1987). *Job tenure, lifetime work interruption, and wage differentials* (Survey of Income and Program Participation, Working Paper No. 8711). Washington, DC: U.S. Bureau of the Census.
Moffitt, R. (1992). Incentive effects of the U.S. welfare system. A review. *Journal of Economic Literature, 30,* 1-61.
Nock, S. (2001). The marriages of equally dependent spouses. *Journal of Family Issues, 22,* 755-775.
Ozawa, M. N. (1997). Demographic changes and their implications. In M. Reisch & E. Gambrill (Eds.), *Social work in the 21st century* (pp. 8-27). Thousand Oaks, CA: Pine Forge Press.
Ozawa, M. N., & Hong, B. E. (2000). The economic impact of widowhood, divorce, and separation on nonaged women. *Journal of Social Policy and Social Work, 2,* 5-17.
Ozawa, M. N., & Hong, B. E. (undated). The effects of EITC and children's allowances on the economic well-being of children: Family size as a policy issue. St. Louis, MO: George Warren Brown School of Social Work Washington University.
Ozawa, M. N., & Wang, Y. T. (1993). The effects of children and education on women's earnings history. *Social Work Research, 22,* 14-30.
Plotnick, R. D. (1995). Income distribution. In *Encyclopedia of social work* (pp. 1439-1447). Washington, DC: NASW Press.
Smith, J. P. (1989). Women, mothers, and work. In M. N. Ozawa (Ed.), *Women's life cycle and economic insecurity: Problems and proposals* (pp. 42-70). Westport, CT: Greenwood Press, 1989.
Smith, J. P., & Ward, M. (1989). Women in the labor market and women in the family. *Journal of Economic Perspectives, 3,* 9-23.
Solomon, C. D. (1992). Aid to families with dependent children (AFDC): Need standards, payment standards, and maximum benefits. *CRS Report for Congress* (93)-63 EPW). Washington, DC: Congressional Research Service.
Social Security Administration. (2000). *Annual statistical supplement, 2000, to the Social Security Bulletin.* Washington, DC: Author.
Triest, R. K. (1990). The effect of income taxation on labor supply in the United States. *Journal of Human Resources, 25,* 491-516.
U.S. Bureau of the Census. (1984a). *Current population survey: Annual demographic file, 1970* (ICPSR 7561) (2nd ICPSR ed.). Ann Arbor, MI: Inter-University Consortium for Political and Social Research.
U.S. Bureau of the Census. (1984b). *Current population survey: Annual demographic file, 1980* (ICPSR 8040) (2nd ICPSR ed.). Ann Arbor, MI: Inter-University Consortium for Political and Social Research.
U.S. Bureau of the Census. (1991). *Current population survey: Annual demographic file, 1990* (ICPSR 9475) (2nd ICPSR ed.). Ann Arbor, MI: Inter-University Consortium for Political and Social Research.
U.S. Bureau of the Census. (2000a). *Current population survey: Annual demographic file, 2000* (ICPSR 3048) (2nd ICPSR ed.). Ann Arbor, MI: Inter-University Consortium for Political and Social Research.
U.S. Bureau of the Census. (2000b). *Statistical abstract of the United States: 2000.* Washington, DC: Author.

U.S. Bureau of the Census. (2001). *Historical income tables–Households* [on-line]. Available: (*http://www.census.gov/hhes/income/histinc/h09a.html*).

Wood, R. G., Corcoran, M. E., & Courant, P. En. (1993). Pay differences among the highly paid: The male-female earnings gap in lawyers' salaries. *Journal of Labor Economics*, 11, 417-441.

Central Appalachia–
Still the *Other* America

Susan Sarnoff

SUMMARY. This paper celebrates the 40th anniversary of the publication of Michael Harrington's *The Other America*, which is recognized as a critical catalyst to the development of the War on Poverty. It focuses on Harrington's observations about Central Appalachia, noting the degree to which the characteristics Harrington observed in 1962 persist there these forty years later. *[Article copies available for a fee from The Haworth Document Delivery Service: 1-800-HAWORTH. E-mail address: <docdelivery@haworthpress.com> Website: <http://www.HaworthPress.com> © 2003 by The Haworth Press, Inc. All rights reserved.]*

KEYWORDS. Poverty, Appalachia, Harrington, *The Other America*

INTRODUCTION

When Michael Harrington (1962) wrote *The Other America*, he addressed "poverty amid plenty" in many parts of the country. Perhaps no area that he discussed, however, received as much attention as Appalachia.

Harrington noted that Appalachian poverty is unusual in ways that challenge many deeply held beliefs about poverty in America. Appala-

---

Susan Sarnoff, MSW, DSW, is Assistant Professor, Ohio University, Department of Social Work, Morton Hall 522, Athens, OH 45701 (E-mail: sarnoff@ohio.edu).

[Haworth co-indexing entry note]: "Central Appalachia–Still the *Other* America." Sarnoff, Susan. Co-published simultaneously in *Journal of Poverty* (The Haworth Press, Inc.) Vol. 7, No. 1/2, 2003, pp. 123-139; and: *Rediscovering the Other America: The Continuing Crisis of Poverty and Inequality in the United States* (ed: Keith M. Kilty, and Elizabeth A. Segal) The Haworth Press, Inc., 2003, pp. 123-139. Single or multiple copies of this article are available for a fee from The Haworth Document Delivery Service [1-800-HAWORTH, 9:00 a.m. - 5:00 p.m. (EST). E-mail address: docdelivery@haworthpress.com].

chian poverty does not seem to result from discrimination based on minority status, emanate from recent immigrants' inability to assimilate into American culture, or reflect a rejection of traditional American norms and values.

Harrington observed two additional characteristics of Appalachian poverty that made it particularly unusual–and unusually intractable. He first pointed out that the long-term, unmitigated poverty typical of Appalachia, which persists in times that are economically beneficial for most Americans, is particularly demoralizing because it destroys aspirations. This type of poverty, which affords little escape through education or innovation, leaves people unable to take advantage of those opportunities that do become available. Second, Harrington noted that people raised in Appalachia were viewed as unfit for urban life, because it was assumed that their acculturation, values, education and training failed to prepare them to adapt to a rapidly changing, highly technological, urban America. Yet he also noted that Appalachians were often forced to choose between leaving their environments or risking lifelong poverty. This has changed little since Harrington's writing, because employment availability in Central Appalachia has changed little since then.

Harrington also pointed out that poverty that exists amid plenty renders the poor invisible. People do not expect others to be poor when they are not; consequently, they do not perceive these poor, whether they are isolated in inner cities or remote rural regions.

Since his writing, the "culture of poverty" perspective that Harrington credited as the cause of Appalachian poverty has been criticized as victim-blaming by some. Blee and Billings (2000), however, observe that this is the case only if individuals are blamed, and that the "culture of poverty" accurately reflects the systemic nature of poverty.

Harrington's description of Appalachian poverty and its causes and manifestation, resonates even these 40 years after its publication, particularly in regard to Central Appalachia, suggesting not only that it was accurate then, but also that circumstances have not changed considerably since. In fact, Appalachia has been compared to the Third World (Lohman, 1990; Reid, undated; Sarnoff, 2001) and to a colony (Blauner, 1969); and VISTA, a domestic parallel to the Peace Corps, was created to serve the region (Lewis and Billings, 1997).

This paper will review Harrington's observations about Central Appalachia, noting the degree to which the characteristics he observed persist there 40 years since the beginning of the War on Poverty, which *The Other America* helped to spawn. It will take its outline from the aspects of Harrington's observations noted above, comparing them to today's Central Appalachia to demonstrate how little has changed, and offer some insights about why this is the case.

WHO ARE THE CENTRAL APPALACHIAN POOR?

The poor of Central Appalachia, in Harrington's time and today, share many characteristics with the most affluent Americans: they tend to be white, largely of Anglo-Saxon ethnicity, Protestant, and trace their roots in America back many generations (Duncan, 1999). Cunningham (1991) noted, however, that most white Appalachians are of Celtic, or Scottish-Irish-Welsh, origin, and although those groups are considered "WASPs" by American standards, they have long been exploited minorities in Great Britain, to which the continued strife in Northern Ireland and its unquestioned inclusion in the Third World attest. As a result, elite Americans of English derivation have always viewed them as inferiors. Cunningham also pointed out that many of these "inferiors" were brought to this country against their will as forced labor, prisoners or debtors. In this way, white Appalachians share histories that are often closer to those of African-American slaves than of other white immigrants–they were brought against their will, without family, property, prospects or preparation for the changes they would face in this country.

Since the 1960s, poverty in the United States has also been associated with female-headed families. Yet, while intact families remain far more common in Appalachia than elsewhere in the United States (Rural and Appalachian Youth and Family Consortium, 1996), they are also more likely to be poor than intact families elsewhere in the country (Rogers, Mencken and Mencken, 1997).

As a result, Central Appalachians do not fit the stereotype that most Americans have of poor people in this country (non-white, foreign-born or part of single-parent families). Yet Central Appalachia has long had, and continues to have, substandard public schools, corrupt political institutions and limited infrastructure more commonly associated with poor people that fit the stereotype (Duncan, 1992 and 1999; Fitchen, 1998).

According to Stock (1996), the first Europeans who settled in Appalachia were farmers and small producers who felt alienated from other Americans from the time the Constitution was ratified, believing that that document favored merchants and speculators. These settlers became more anti-authoritarian and anti-tax as their occasional requests for legislation favorable to their interests, such as rights to move products down the Mississippi River, were ignored. These early European-American

Appalachians believed that eastern elites most benefitted from government policies, and therefore, should provide the bulk of support for them. Eastern elites, on the other hand, argued that luxuries such as whiskey should absorb the bulk of heavy taxation–not understanding that many mountaineers produced small amounts of whiskey (locally known as "moonshine") because it could be stored or marketed more easily than their other products, and often substituted for cash on the frontier. The Whiskey Rebellion was the result of this impasse (Stock, 1996).

Despite their traditional reluctance to rely on government, since the Depression a major source of Appalachian income has come from public benefit programs. Need for these benefits is inevitable given the extent of mining and other work-related injuries, and environmental hazards to which Appalachians have been exposed (Duncan, 1999). Also inevitable are disabilities from birth or early childhood caused by poor nutrition and inadequate prenatal care, which are also more common in Appalachia than elsewhere in the U.S. (Rural and Appalachian Youth and Family Consortium, 1996). Evidence exists that some Appalachians become resigned to accepting disability payments as a way of life, and sometimes welcome them at least for their regularity (Erikson, 1976). This even leads some to encourage labeling of their children as disabled to ensure that they will qualify for lifelong benefits (Janofsky, 1998).

It is difficult to imagine that the antebellum image of Appalachia was romanticized for its traditionalism. Post-Civil War attempts to unify the nation, however, identified Appalachian "difference" as threatening the then-new ideal of American homogeneity (Shapiro, 1978). It was not until the end of the 19th century, when lumber and coal companies sought to exploit Appalachia's natural resources, however, that the image of the "ignorant hillbilly" took shape (Rolland, 1999; Shapiro, 1978).

While the civil rights movement improved the image of African-American Appalachians after the 1950s, it superimposed yet another stereotype on that of the white "hillbilly": that of the provincial mountain white, or "redneck" (yet another inaccuracy, since the term redneck originated in union organizers' self-identification by wearing red neckerchiefs). While some Southern white Appalachians did agitate to thwart integration of the races and classes during the civil rights movement, any Appalachians who fought to maintain their traditional rurality were erroneously assumed to be doing so out of prejudice. In reality, when Appalachians are viewed as opposing "progress," it is because much of what has been offered to them as progress has resulted, instead, in personal and environmental exploitation.

WHY DOES CENTRAL APPALACHIAN POVERTY PERSIST?

Northern and Southern Appalachia have become considerably less poor over the past 40 years, while Central Appalachia has remained economically much as it was prior to the War on Poverty ("Appalachia: Hollow Promises," 1999; "Shrinking Appalachia," 1999). This occurred as a result of civil rights era targeting of benefits and services to minorities; the Student Nonviolent Coordinating Committee's (SNCC) and the Congress on Racial Equality's (CORE) greater success in organizing minorities in urban ghettoes, particularly in the north (Chalmers, 1996); and the Appalachian Regional Commission's identification of "growth centers" promising for industry, none of which existed in Central Appalachia (Drake, 2001). In fact, most of Appalachia has continued to be poorer than the rest of the United States since, and despite, the War on Poverty. However, Farmer (undated) noted that the poorest counties of Central Appalachia continue to have poverty rates three times those of other poor counties in the country; and the Rural and Appalachian Youth and Family Consortium (1996) observed that the area continues to have unemployment rates that are twice the national average.

The persistence of Central Appalachian poverty is extreme by another dimension: the majority of residents have been poor for a much longer period of time than have residents of inner cities, suburban rust belts or midwestern farm families in the United States (Arcury and Porter, 1985). Many poor urban communities in the United States serve as temporary stopping points for new immigrants, students, or newly single parents, who move away once they acquire skills or savings, so the regions remain poor while their residents change. Central Appalachian populations, instead, have tended to remain poor in place for many generations (Adams and Duncan, 1992).

A BRIEF HISTORY OF CENTRAL APPALACHIAN POVERTY

Since the Civil War, the history of Central Appalachia has been one of exploitation: of land and other natural resources, and especially of people. By the end of the 19th century, lumber companies were clear-cutting huge areas of Appalachia, using corruption, intimidation and legal subterfuges to ignore property owners' rights, unless those property owners were willing to sell their land or the trees on their land for a fraction of their value. This not only depleted the area of timber, but also caused erosion, which depleted most of the fertile soil from the area (Shannon,

1981). Coal companies, in turn, early in the 20th century, bought land "rights" from the lumber companies after the trees were gone. They expanded further by offering to buy only the mineral rights to properties still held by local landowners, then driving the owners off the land in a variety of ways: buying it for a fraction of its value, as the lumber companies had done; forging sale documents; and even murdering unyielding landowners and buying out their widows (Gaventa, 1978; Wright, 1978; Erikson, 1976).

While the lumber companies employed some local residents, the coal companies required much larger workforces. By paying low wages they forced families to allow young children to work beside their fathers, and sometimes their mothers (Bettman, 1974). They also imported workers from outside Central Appalachia, hiring mixes of former black sharecroppers and immigrants, in part to create dissension among workers (Arcury and Porter, 1985). However, Central Appalachians tended to view others who shared common values as equals, respect others who chose mountain life, and have a long tradition of intermarriage with both escaped slaves and Indians (Williams, 1985). As a result, they had no difficulty organizing with this diverse workforce for improved working conditions (which came as a result of unionization). They even overcame language barriers to organize with immigrants who spoke no English.

Only later, when the coal companies stepped up their efforts to create dissension among miners in response to early attempts to unionize, using African-Americans as scabs (Murolo and Chitty 2001) and favoring white workers with better housing and jobs (creating class warfare among groups of the poor to offset anger against the rich owners) did segregationist attitudes develop among whites in the Central and Northern regions of Appalachia (Williams, 1985). Interracial marriage was then discouraged, and one reason that Central Appalachia now appears to have few minorities is that even those Appalachians with African-American or American Indian ancestors may deny or be unaware of that fact.

Still, at the beginning of the 20th century, when most unions were segregated, United Mine Workers (UMW) membership was 20% African-American. This meant that fully two-thirds of African-American union members belonged to the UMW, making it the most racially inclusive union of its time (Murolo and Chitty, 2001).

Despite the coal companies' exploitation, coal mining has always been a costly business with a small profit margin. To keep salaries low and increase profits, coal companies began as total institutions, building housing, roads and schools, operating company stores and hiring company doctors. Not only did this keep down salaries, taxes and other operating costs, it also ensured that "public" services would meet the companies' needs–and some actually generated profits. They also allowed the companies to exert extensive control over workers: strikers were driven from their homes and denied medical care; widows and orphans were quickly evicted, lessening reminders of the dangers of mining; and once indebted to the company store, miners were forced at gunpoint to remain in the coal camps until they worked off what they owed or died trying. The latter result was more likely, particularly in light of the "creative bookkeeping" typically performed on company store accounts (Gaventa, 1978).

The coal companies were able to maintain great control because only a small number of individuals and corporations owned most of the land and industry. This also enabled them to keep taxes, particularly those related to the coal industry, extremely low (Barkan and Lloyd, 1970; Diehl, 1970; Kirby, 1969; Walls, 1968-69; Blizzard, 1966), and to control politics, as well (Batteau, 1990). For instance, Corbin (1981) noted that from 1888 until 1924, all of Kentucky's governors were either coal company officials or their lackeys. This was exacerbated by the fact that coal was particularly vital to the nation's economy from the mid-1800s through the mid-1900s. Devaluation of local residents and the importance of coal to the national economy also enabled owners to use the government against striking miners, as in the infamous Matewan Massacre (Scott, 1995) and the Battle of Blair Mountain, two major union battles quashed by federal troops, the latter the only instance in which the federal government bombed its own citizens (Lee, 1969).

This history offers clues to the persistence of Appalachian poverty. For one, Appalachians have never been viewed as deserving of a share of the "American Dream." Instead, they have been treated as others–outsiders in their own country, undeserving of benefits because they fail to conform to American stereotypes. Antipoverty programs are often designed so outsiders are ineligible for benefits, or are forced to conform to externally imposed standards (giving up traditions, leaving family members) to gain eligibility. The persistence of Appalachian poverty throughout the lumbering and mining years also demonstrates that industrialization alone is no economic panacea (Haynes, 1997).

CENTRAL APPALACHIANS AND GOVERNMENT MISTRUST

Mistrust of government only exacerbates the lack of fit between programs and those who could benefit from them (if their benefits and eligibility factors were redesigned). Learned distrust of government has had long-term effects on Appalachia. Cynthia Duncan's (1999) study contrasting life in New England with that of Appalachian Kentucky and Mississippi identified how New England town meetings encouraged open government, civic involvement, shared resources and egalitarian social structures. In contrast, she showed that in both Southern and Central Appalachia, small groups of elites control government and public employment, hoarding scarce resources. Duncan demonstrated that failure to provide adequate public services, including roads, schools and jobs, reflected not only limited resources, but corruption and lack of social concern as well. She also observed that while race is used to demarcate "haves" from "have nots" in Southern Appalachia, family names and reputations serve the same function in Central Appalachia. Politics also have been responsible for inequitable carving up of poverty funds, so a few sections of Appalachia, represented by powerful legislators, have received more than their share of anti-poverty resources, while areas with less powerful or less concerned representatives fall further behind ("Appalachia: Hollow Promises," 1999).

Another contrast between Central and Southern Appalachia is that Southern Appalachians, while mistrusting local government as much as Central Appalachians, have been substantially assisted by the federal government during, and since, the civil rights movement. Ironically, funds targeted to minorities have helped not only them, but all residents of communities that receive minority-targeted funds. As a result, Southern Appalachians are not as distrustful of all levels of government as are Central Appalachians.

Such distrust has long-lasting effects. For instance, West Virginia is currently facing a major threat to its already meager medical infrastructure. While some insurers are refusing coverage to medical practitioners in the state, because juries tend to approve some of the highest malpractice payouts in that state (Tranum, 2001), others are charging such high premiums that practitioners are choosing to move their practices out of the state (Clines, 2002). Attempts at tort reform are not unique to Central Appalachia, but its history of worker exploitation has made citizens reluctant to trust the testimony of medical practitioners and unusually sympathetic toward injured workers.

WHY WILL APPALACHIANS NOT URBANIZE?

The Appalachian poor have tended to remain rural, while anti-poverty programs have targeted their services to the urban poor. This targeting strategy assumes not only that the poor are worse off in urban communities, but also that the best opportunity to escape poverty is to relocate to urban areas, which presumably have more available jobs. Ironically, unskilled manufacturing jobs have diminished everywhere, but particularly in urban areas.

Policymakers generally study urban poverty, and often fail to understand its rural counterpart. For instance, in urban areas home and vehicle ownership are signs of affluence, as there is considerable rental housing and the availability of public transportation makes owning a vehicle a luxury. Rural areas often have limited rental property, because housing costs are low, although housing may be substandard, access to potable water and other services may be costly or unreliable if available at all, and roads, schools and other infrastructure may suffer from insufficient tax bases and limited support for improvements. In rural areas, too, public transportation is minimal if not nonexistent. Yet poor rural residents may be denied various forms of assistance solely because they are land owners; they also may be assumed able to travel to distant jobs because they own a vehicle, although the vehicle may be in poor repair, or may be a farm vehicle, such as a tractor.

Browne (2001) posits that policymakers assume that people live in rural areas by choice, because the rural areas that those policymakers know best are bucolic, resource-rich seasides, ski areas and other vacation places, rather than the rural areas the poor inhabit. Browne further notes that the nation has limited rural policy, assuming that farm policy assists all rural residents and that relocation is always an option for the rural poor.

WHY IS CENTRAL APPALACHIAN POVERTY NOT MORE VISIBLE?

To further complicate circumstances, the geography of Central Appalachia is a challenge to the best construction engineers. Frequent flooding (exacerbated by the dumping of mining by-products in local waterways) and mountains and hollows that are naturally difficult to traverse and pave render commuting to jobs in nearby cities difficult. This forces residents to choose between leaving the familiarity and safety of home (as many young people have done) or foregoing opportunities for economic advancement ("Appalachia: Hollow Promises," 1999).

Such geographic isolation has proved attractive to only a few industries, specifically those that benefit from clandestine operation. Hence the stereotype "moonshiner" and the far more insidious use of the hollows and streams for the dumping of environmental hazards (Caudill, 1962). In fact, some flooding, such as that which occurred at Buffalo Creek in 1972 (Erikson, 1976), was actually caused by environmental dumping that raised riverbeds so much that they could no longer accommodate rainwater.

The people who own land in environmentally unsound areas do so because they have limited choices. They cannot gain enough from the sale of their land to buy elsewhere, so selling means giving up land ownership. Antipoverty programs do little to help these people, since urban-centric policymakers do not perceive land ownership as important to economic well-being.

DOES CENTRAL APPALACHIA REFLECT A "CULTURE OF POVERTY"?

Oscar Lewis's (1966) familiar construct of a "culture of poverty" was invoked by Harrington to explain the persistence of poverty in Appalachia. However, the culture of poverty, as Lewis defined it, has been discredited as discriminatory and victim blaming. The preceding discussion of the history and politics of Appalachia suggests that attitudes that may appear to reflect indifference may instead result from actual experience with uncaring or corrupt officials and policies that have failed to produce what they promised. The "culture of poverty" implies that the poor are lazy and unwilling to work. However, Blee and Billings (1986) have shown that Appalachians' attitudes about work can be better understood as a form of resistance to the separation of work and control enforced by mine owners and other exploitative employers. They later added that "culture of poverty" constructs are useful in demonstrating that rural Appalachian poverty is systemic rather than individual (Billings & Blee, 2000).

Human capital theory, which explains income variations as resulting from productivity differences (DiNitto, 2000), may be supported by Appalachian poverty, but with qualification. What Halperin (1996) has defined as "the Kentucky Way" is a form of economic resistance not to capitalism, but to dependence on capitalism. Owning even a small amount of "hardscrabble" land acts as a buffer against reliance on others or on the market economy, permitting subsistence farming, cash crops and hunting and fishing for food. Remaining near family provides support in hard times that lessens reliance on government programs. In this context, the refusal to adapt to such modern concepts as relocating for advanced education or career opportunities or going into debt to maintain a lifestyle beyond one's means can be seen as a functional strategy, albeit that it ill prepares family members who might prefer a different way of life.

Another factor that relates to the "Kentucky Way" is that of the informal labor market (White and Marks, 1999). One way that Appalachians have adapted to frequent unemployment and underemployment has been to use periods of joblessness or inadequate earning to create crafts, raise subsistence crops, catch fish and meat, gather naturally growing herbs such as black cohosh and ginseng, and chop wood for personal use and sale. In this context, it is easy to understand "moonshining," and its newer counterpart, marijuana growing, as alternative income sources, favored because there are always markets for these products. That such activity is illegal is not its attraction, but illegality is less of a deterrent to people in desperate economic circumstances, particularly when those people's views of government are far from benign.

This is a less frequently identified reason that many Appalachians eschew leaving home or seeking careers that require extensive preparation: this wide variety of income sources, and familiarity with local markets, while not guaranteeing high incomes, does increase economic options. Such an array of options are particularly useful when the economy is weak–and the Central Appalachian economy has been weak even when the broader economy has been strong. In fact, while well-intentioned economists, legislators and community activists often decry the increase in low-paying service sector jobs, these jobs are often welcomed by Appalachians precisely because they fit into the constellation of income opportunities that can be taken advantage of as needed without long-term commitments.

One of the most devastating social effects of the Appalachian stereotype has been the internalization of a sense of inferiority (Rolland, 1999) which is clearly unwarranted in view of the facts. Such inferiority, however, can hold people back not only from externally imposed "progress," but from daring to fulfill personal ambitions, whatever they might be. This sense can only be overcome by changing the social landscape, enabling citizens to see "their own kind" succeed without giving up their traditions and cultural connections. Even when the social landscape has changed, however, there is an understandable lag time until people recognize that change, and until they believe that it will persist. In the meantime, people have to choose between cultural adaptations toward "progress" and those that maintain group solidarity (Jones, 1997).

In Central Appalachia, pronunciation and word usage, or dialect, separate insiders and outsiders. Some words are purposely not pronounced as they are spelled to identify outsiders, with the word "Appalachia" itself serving as an example of this. ("Insiders" pronounce Appalachia with a short third "a.") These facts suggest that theories attributing poverty to exploitation and social structure are most strongly supported by the reality of Appalachian poverty.

CENTRAL APPALACHIA TODAY

"Progress" in Appalachia today takes many forms, including continued exploitation in the forms of strip mining and other environmental devastation and attempts to impose modernization by replacing public benefits with job training and placement without regard to personal interests, aptitudes or job locations. It also takes the form of relocating jobs from Appalachia to places outside of the United States, where environmental standards are lower and workers less able to organize for improved pay and working conditions (Mittal, 2000).

These facts leave Central Appalachians worse off than they were in the past, when at least the mining industry relied on Central Appalachian workers. When coal was depleted from an area, coal companies moved on, leaving roads and buildings to fall into disrepair (McKelvey, 1968). In some places, mine owners went so far as to tear up railroad track that they had installed before they left, rather than leave this meager bit of infrastructure for their former employees. Lacking not only adequate infrastructure, but also natural resources, investment capital, entrepreneurial experience and a significant tax base, efforts to rebuild communities often foundered. In fact, many portions of Central Appalachia still lack adequate roads or pure water ("Appalachia: Hollow Promises," 1999). Worse than this meager legacy, the coal and lumber barons left behind distrust of all capitalists and government activities (Gaventa, 1978; Erikson, 1976).

Ironically, however, Central Appalachians love their land more than typically mobile Americans, and stay in spite of these problems. In fact, the greatest resource of Central Appalachia is its residents. They deserve–finally–a form of progress compatible with their needs and interests.

Such progress would encourage land ownership, not penalize it. It would create employment opportunities compatible with the area and its people: building on indigenous talents such as quilting, woodworking, and crafts; and would pro-rate benefits for part-time work, recognizing that most Appalachians work full-time, but at more than one job.

Progress can involve citizens in planning compatible economic development (Dunbar, 1999). This is the only strategy that can result in long-term success for all involved, a strategy that requires recognizing that residents' knowledge of and dedication to their region is an invaluable resource. By linking this knowledge of historic, cultural and natural resources, Appalachians are in many instances identifying economic alternatives that are compatible with natural resource protection. They do not need ideas about these imposed from outside–in fact, attempts to offer them consistently fail; but they do need technical assistance to help secure funding and develop skills residents identify as lacking.

For instance, successful businesses have developed in Central Appalachia in recent years built on traditions that are gaining appeal outside of the area: growing specialty crops incompatible with agribusiness, medicinal herbs in particular; creating and marketing packaged specialty foods and crafts; and developing recreational activities that appeal to nature lovers and sports enthusiasts (such as hiking, climbing, rowing, hunting and fishing). Two major initiatives, Rural Action and the Appalachian Cooperative Exchange Network (ACEnet), offer a wide range of activities that support local home- and farm-based businesses. In one such initiative, Rural Action teaches farmers about alternative crops. And ACEnet, among other things, operates a professional kitchen which is time-shared by local small businesses wishing to package their products for broader distribution (Prigoff, 2000). A university-based small business incubator assists local businesses to develop and market new products and services, and to learn the skills needed for such expansion.

THE FUTURE OF CENTRAL APPALACHIA

These activities can lead to additional business opportunities. For instance, the need to restock depleted rivers has led to the development of trout and catfish hatcheries; and the rough terrain, reminiscent of the Scottish highlands, is a natural site for golf courses. Ohio has recently invested millions of dollars in the restoration of buildings that were part of the Underground Railroad, to preserve the state's history and encourage tourism. Increased tourism will, in turn, increase the demand for hotels, restaurants, campgrounds and craft shops.

Ironically, too, Appalachia has recently become "fashionable." The success of the commercial film *O Brother, Where Art Thou?* has generated renewed interest in bluegrass music, which is indigenous to the area. Similarly, the reluctance of many Americans to fly since the recent terrorist attacks may increase interest in more local vacation areas.

Two recent investors in Central Appalachia have been journalist Terry Anderson, who used some of the compensation he received for the years he was a hostage in Beirut to set up a foundation for Appalachian advancement and to open a blues club and Cajun restaurant in Athens, Ohio; and Hot Tuna guitarist Jorma Kaukonen, who created a guitar camp in Darwin, Ohio. The latter has been so successful that it has spawned a gourmet restaurant, a concert theater and a syndicated public radio show, *Live from Fur Peace Ranch*.

Social work has been extremely remiss in failing to recognize the needs of people in rural areas. Clearly, Central Appalachians fit all of the characteristics of a minority group, but they are recognized as a minority group as a matter of law only in the city of Cincinnati. Others continue to perceive "hillbillies" as ignorant and backward, rather than as members of a unique and traditional culture that deserves to be respected and preserved.

Central Appalachia, like so much of rural America, missed out on much of what Toffler defined as "second wave" infrastructure development (Toffler, 1980). In some ways, however, this could be advantageous as society develops "third wave" technology. Paved highways are less necessary as the information superhighway largely replaces it. And increasingly, workers are escaping urban areas as they have more freedom to travel–not only for leisure, but to transport their workplaces anywhere they can operate their laptops. Such workers seek traditional communities that afford scenic views and nearby recreation, both of which are plentiful in Central Appalachia. To attract telecommuters, however, communities must offer high standards of public elementary and secondary education and public services, which Central Appalachia is lacking. If Central Appalachia can accommodate these workers' infrastructure needs, they can become appealing workplaces indeed, having preserved so much of the tradition and rurality that people have always sought, but long considered incompatible with career success. Success is, of course, far from guaranteed.

In the meantime, Central Appalachia, while having moved from its 1960-era level of poverty (more due to public benefits than to industry) still lags behind the rest of the country economically, much as it did at Harrington's writing. Therefore, Central Appalachia has, for the most part, not entered the mainstream of America, and is, instead, still very much the "other" America.

BIBLIOGRAPHY

Adams, Terry K. and Greg J. Duncan. (1992) "Long-term poverty in rural areas," in Duncan, Cynthia R., ed. *Rural Poverty in America*. NY: Auburn House, 63-93.

"Appalachia: hollow promises" (1999) *Columbus Dispatch*, September 26-29.

Arcury, Thomas A. and Julia D. Porter. (1985) "Household composition in appalachian kentucky in 1900," *Journal of Family History*, Summer, 183-195.

Barkan, Barry and R. Baldwin Lloyd. (1970) "Picking poverty's pocket," *Article One*, 1, 2, May, 21-29.

Batteau, Allen W. (1990) *The invention of appalachia*. Tucson, AZ: University of Arizona Press.

Bettmann, Otto L. (1974) *The good old days–they were terrible!* NY: Random House.

Billings, Dwight and Kathleen Blee. (2000) *The road to poverty: the making of wealth and hardship in appalachia*. NY: Cambridge University Press.

Blauner, Robert. (1969) "Internal colonialism and ghetto revolt," *Social Problems*, 16, 4, Spring, 393-498.

Blee, Kathleen and Dwight Billings. (1986) "Reconstructing daily life in the past: an hermeneutical approach to ethnographic data," *Sociological Quarterly*, 27, 443-62.

Blizzard, William C. (1966) "West virginia wonderland," *Appalachian South*, Summer.

Browne, William P. (2001) The failure of national rural policy. Washington, DC: Georgetown University Press.

Caudill, Harry M. (1962) *Night comes to the cumberlands*. Boston: Little, Brown & Co.

Chalmers, David. (1996) *And the crooked places made straight: the struggle for social change in the 1960s*, second edition. Baltimore, Johns Hopkins University Press.

Clines, Francis X. (2002) "Insurance-squeezed doctors folding tents in west virginia," *New York Times*, June 13.

Corbin, David. (1981) *Life, work and rebellion in the coal fields*. Urbana, IL: University of Illinois Press.

Cunningham, Rodger. (1991) *Apples on the flood*. Knoxville, TN: University of Tennessee Press.

Diehl, Richard. (1970) "How international energy elite rules," *Peoples' Appalachia*, March.

DiNitto, Diana M. (2000) *Social policy: politics & public policy*. Boston: Allyn & Bacon.

Drake, Richard B. (2001) *A history of appalachia*. Lexington, KY: The University Press of Kentucky.

Dunbar, Ellen Russell. (1999) "Strengthening services in rural communities through blended funding," in Carlton-LaNey, Iris B., Richard L. Edwards and P. Nelson Reid, *Preserving and Strengthening Small Towns and Rural Communities*. Washington, DC: NASW Press, 15-26.

Duncan, Cynthia M. (1992) "Persistent poverty in appalachia: scarce work and rigid stratification," in Duncan, Cynthia M., ed. *Rural Poverty in America*. NY: Auburn House, 111-133.

Duncan, Cynthia M. (1999) *Worlds apart: why poverty persists in rural america*. New Haven, CT: Yale University Press.

Erikson, Kai T. (1976) *Everything in its path*. NY: Simon & Schuster.

Farmer, Suzanne Minichillo. (undated) "Observations and recommendations for distressed appalachian counties" [online at University of Kentucky Appalachian Center website].
Fitchen, Janet M. (1998) "Rural poverty and rural social work," in Ginsburg, Leon, ed. *Social Work in Communities, third edition*. Alexandria, VA: Council on Social Work Education, 115-134.
Gaventa, John. (1978) "Property, coal & theft," in Lewis, Helen Matthews, Linda Johnson and Donald Askins, eds., *Colonialism in Modern America: An Appalachian Case*. Boone, NC: Appalachian Consortium Press, 141-159.
Halperin, Rhoda H. (1996) "Rethinking the informal economy: implications for regional analysis," *Research in Economic Anthropology*, 17, 43-79.
Haynes, Ada F. (1997) *Poverty in central appalachia*. NY: Garland Publishing, Inc.
Janofsky, Michael. (1998) "Pessimism retains grip on appalachian poor." *New York Times*, February 9.
Jones, Patricia Smith. (1997) "Dialect as a deterrent to cultural stripping: why appalachian migrants continue to talk that talk," *Journal of Appalachian Studies*, 3, 2, 253-261.
Kirby, Richard. (1969) "Kentucky coal: owners, taxes and profits," *Appalachian Lookout*, 1, 6, October, 19-27.
Lee, Howard. (1969) *Bloodletting in america*. Morgantown, WV: West Virginia University.
Lewis, Oscar. (1966) "The culture of poverty," *Scientific American*, 215, 19-25.
Lewis, Ronald L. and Dwight D. Billings. (1997) "Appalachian culture and economic development: a retrospective view on the theory and literature," *Journal of Appalachian Studies*, 3, 1, 3-42.
Lohman, R. A. (1990) "Four perspectives on appalachian culture and poverty," *Journal of the Appalachian Studies Association*, 2, 76-88.
McKelvey, V. E. (1968) "Appalachia: problems and opportunities," *Geological Survey Professional Paper 580*. Washington, DC: U.S. Geological Survey.
Mittal, Anuradha. (2000) "The south in the north," *Views from the South*. Chicago: Food First.
Murolo, Priscilla and A. B. Chitty. (2001) *From the folks who brought you the weekend*. NY: The New Press.
Prigoff, Arlene. (2000) *Economics for social workers*. Scarborough, Ont.: Wadsworth, Thomson.
Reid, Herbert teaches a course for the Appalachian Center at the University of Kentucky. *www.uky.edu/RGS/AppalCenter*.
Rolland, Susanne Mosteller. (1999) "Valuing rural community: appalachian social work students' perspectives on faculty attitudes toward their culture," in Carlton-LaNey, Iris B., Richard L. Edwards and P. Nelson Reid, *Preserving and Strengthening Small Towns and Rural Communities*. Washington, DC: NASW Press, 326-334.
Rogers, Cynthia, Kimberly Mencken and F. Carson Mencken. (1997) "Female labor force participation in central appalachia: a descriptive analysis," *Journal of Appalachian Studies*, 3, 2.
Rural and Appalachian Youth and Family Consortium. (1996) "Parenting practices and interventions among marginalized families in appalachia: building on family strengths," *Family Relations*, October, 387-396.
Sarnoff, Susan K. (2001) "Appalachia as a third world region: what can be learned," *27th Annual Third World Conference*, Chicago, IL, March 23.

Scott, Shaunna L. (1995) *Two sides of everything: the cultural construction of class consciousness in harlan county, ky.* Albany, NY: State University of New York Press.

Shannon, Irwin. (1981) *Southeastern ohio in depression and war: the disintegration of an area.* Columbus, OH: Ohio State University.

Shapiro, Henry David. (1978) *Appalachia on our mind: the southern mountains and mountaineers in the american consciousness, 1870-1920.* Chapel Hill, NC: University of North Carolina Press.

"Shrinking appalachia" (1999) *New York Times*, June 11.

Stock, Catherine McNicol. (1996) *Rural radicals.* NY: Cornell University Press.

Toffler, Alvin. (1980) *The third wave.* NY: Morrow.

Tranum, Sam. (2001) "Medical malpractice facts in dispute," *Charleston Daily Mail*, November 26.

Walls, David. (1968-9) "Research bulletins," issues of *Appalachian Lookout*.

White, Craig and Kathleen Marks. (1999) "A strengths-based approach to rural sustainable development," in Carlton-LaNey, Iris B., Richard L. Edwards and P. Nelson Reid, *Preserving and Strengthening Small Towns and Rural Communities.* Washington, DC: NASW Press, 27-42.

Williams, Leon F. cited in Turner, William H. and Edward J. Cabbell. (1985) *Blacks in america.* Lexington, KY: University Press of Kentucky.

Wright, Warren. (1978) "The big steal," in Lewis, Helen Matthews, Linda Johnson and Donald Askins, eds., *Colonialism in Modern America: An Appalachian Case.* Boone, NC: Appalachian Consortium Press, 161-175.

Welfare Policy, Welfare Participants, and CalWORKS Caseworkers: How Participants Are Informed of Supportive Services

Elizabeth Bartle

Gabriela Segura

SUMMARY. One aspect of the Personal Responsibility and Work Opportunity Reconciliation Act (PRWORA) of 1996 was explored through focus group interviews with public welfare (CalWORKS/TANF) participants in Los Angeles County. Women were asked how they learned about domestic violence, substance abuse, and mental health services from their caseworker in an effort to begin to evaluate implementation of the PRWORA in regards to these supportive services. The results describe how participants are receiving insufficient information, discouraged from seeking services, obtaining assistance from advocates other than caseworkers, and feeling general fear and distrust. Discussion centers on improvements in the system and training for caseworkers. *[Article copies available for a fee from The Haworth Document Delivery Service: 1-800-HAWORTH. E-mail address: <docdelivery@haworthpress.com> Website: <http://www.HaworthPress.com> © 2003 by The Haworth Press, Inc. All rights reserved.]*

Elizabeth Bartle, PhD, is Assistant Professor, Department of Sociology, Social Welfare Option, California State University Northridge, 18111 Nordhoff St., Northridge, CA 91330-8318 (E-mail: elizabeth.e.bartle@csun.edu).

Gabriela Segura is a sociology/social welfare student in the Department of Sociology, Social Welfare Option, California State University Northridge (E-mail: gaby_seg @hotmail.com).

[Haworth co-indexing entry note]: "Welfare Policy, Welfare Participants, and CalWORKS Caseworkers: How Participants Are Informed of Supportive Services." Bartle, Elizabeth, and Gabriela Segura. Co-published simultaneously in *Journal of Poverty* (The Haworth Press, Inc.) Vol. 7, No. 1/2, 2003, pp. 141-161; and: *Rediscovering the Other America: The Continuing Crisis of Poverty and Inequality in the United States* (ed: Keith M. Kilty, and Elizabeth A. Segal) The Haworth Press, Inc., 2003, pp. 141-161. Single or multiple copies of this article are available for a fee from The Haworth Document Delivery Service [1-800-HAWORTH, 9:00 a.m. - 5:00 p.m. (EST). E-mail address: docdelivery@haworthpress.com].

KEYWORDS. PRWORA/TANF policy evaluation, supportive services, domestic violence, substance abuse, mental health, focus group research, caseworkers

When Michael Harrington's *The Other America* (1962) brought to national attention the widespread structural social problems of poverty and inequality in the United States, public welfare policy had just started to attempt to further institutionalize poverty and inequality for poor women. It did this by sanctioning low-wage work in the paid labor force over parenting for welfare participants (see Abramovitz, 1988). Today, 40 years later, "welfare reform" policy, officially called the Personal Responsibility and Work Opportunity Reconciliation Act (PRWORA) of 1996, has not only succeeded in this task but strengthened structural inequality for poor women by officially promoting marriage in addition to work. In many ways, the PRWORA solidified a 40-year effort to "fundamentally change systems of public support" in the United States for families living in poverty in general and for "single-mother families in particular" (Meyers, Han, Waldfogel, Garfinkel, 2001). This paper addresses one of the changes–a renewed policy focus on specific "behavioral" problems that might prevent participants from working, namely screening, assessment, and the provision of supportive services for domestic violence, drug and alcohol abuse, and mental health issues.

Local and national evaluation efforts of the PRWORA have occurred over the past few years. Evaluative studies have been done on issues such as employment, single-mother family income, and poverty (Meyers, Han, Waldfogel, Garfinkel, 2001; Danziger, Corcoran, Danziger, Heflin, 2000; Cancian, Meyer, 2000), but few studies (Brush, 1999; Woolis, 1998; California Institute of Mental Health, 2000; Swigonski, 1996) have focused primarily on evaluating how this supportive service policy has been implemented. Thus, the purpose of this study was to explore how participants of public welfare learned about domestic violence, substance abuse, and mental health services from their welfare caseworkers in an effort to evaluate implementation of the PRWORA in regards to these supportive services.

BACKGROUND: CONTEXT FOR SUPPORTIVE SERVICES IN WELFARE POLICY

The new policy, Personal Responsibility and Work Opportunity Reconciliation Act (PRWORA) of 1996, ended Aid to Families with Dependent Children (AFDC) and led to the establishment of Temporary Aid to Needy Families (TANF). Among other changes, TANF places a focus on marriage. The PRWORA begins with the following value-laden statements:

> (1) Marriage is the foundation of a successful society. 2) Marriage is an essential institution of a successful society that promotes the interests of children. ... The purpose of this part [TANF] is to increase flexibility of states in operating a program designed to–(1) provide assistance to needy families so that children may be cared for in their own homes or in the homes of relatives; (2) end the dependence of needy parents on government benefits by promoting job preparation, work, and marriage; (3) prevent and reduce the incidence of out-of-wedlock pregnancies and established annual numerical goals for preventing and reducing the incidence of these pregnancies; and (4) encourage the formation and maintenance of two-parent families. (Public Law 104-193 as cited in Rose, 2000)

As Rose (2000) states, this focus on marriage indicates a concern about the increase in female-headed families which "led to a new federal initiative: bonuses for reducing the 'illegitimacy ratio,' defined as the ratio of births to unwed mothers divided by total births" (p. 148).

In an effort to implement this policy, the PRWORA replaces "federal responsibility" with state discretion, financing the TANF program through block grants and allowing each state to determine what "behavioral modification" programs they will develop to help achieve the above goals as well as the more commonly stated goal of work in the paid labor force (Rose, 2000).

With the enactment of TANF, new time limits were implemented. Participants of welfare are to receive aid for 24 months consecutively at any one time and there is a maximum lifetime limit of 60 months. States have the option to shorten time limits. When time limits are reached, states can implement a "full family sanction," terminating aid for the entire family. At this time, vouchers are supposed to be distributed as a "safety net" precaution for the children of these families. PRWORA did allow for exemptions to be filed in cases of "extreme hardship." This is applicable for up to 20 percent of the state's caseload (Rose, 2000). Also, states were mandated to have 25% of single adults on the welfare rolls working or in work related activities in 1998. In 2002, the legislation increases the mandate to 50%. If states fail to meet this requirement, they could lose part of their federal block grant (Rose, 2000).

Even after adults leave welfare and go to work many of them continue to live in poverty. This is true because employment positions that are available to participants are low paying (O'Campo & Rojas-Smith, 1998). Families often incur more expenditure during this time as well, for example, childcare and transportation. With increasing emphasis placed on getting women off welfare and into work and marriage, the need for certain supportive services becomes evident (Myers, Bowling, Wen-Jui, Waldfogel, & Garfinkel, 2001). New legislation recognizes that domestic violence, substance abuse and mental health issues act as barriers to achieving and maintaining employment. With this new policy and its resulting legislation, such as the Family Violence Option, workers are now mandated to screen for the need for these services but are not adequately trained to do so.

DOMESTIC VIOLENCE

Due to the recent push of marriage promotion initiatives, domestic violence advocates are concerned that a woman who is a victim of domestic violence might feel the need to stay in or return to an abusive relationship because of the new time limits mandated in the PRWORA. Some advocates say that the PRWORA penalizes women for circumstances that they do not have the power to change (Browne, Salomon, & Bassuk, 1999). Data taken from Bureau of Justice Statistics and the National Family Violence Survey shows there is a higher rate of assault and severe assault for women as well as children living below the federal poverty level. One recent study included 216 housed low-income single-mothers and 220 homeless single mothers in a northeastern city (Worcester Family Research Project, WFRP, as stated in Browne, Salomon, & Bassuk, 1999). Results revealed that about "two-thirds (63%) of both housed and homeless single mothers had as children experienced severe physical assault by parents or other caretakers. About 60% had experienced severe physical violence by an intimate male partner as adults. Nearly one third of all respondents had been severely physically attacked by their current or most recent partner." In addition to the physical attacks, "about one fifth of all women in the sample had been threatened with death by their current or most recent intimate partner." Severe physical violence was defined as "the occurrence of at least one of the following: being kicked; slapped six or more times; bitten or hit with a fist; hit with an object; beaten up; burned or scalded; choked, strangled, or smothered; threatened or assaulted with a knife or gun; or having one's life threatened in some other manner" (Worcester Family Research Project, as stated in Browne, Salomon, & Bassuk, 1999).

Due to the recent changes in our welfare system mandating workers to screen for domestic violence through the Family Violence Option, research examining partner violence against women welfare participants has grown. Prior research documented the high rates of partner violence in the lives of AFDC participants; current research has focused on exploring the relationship between partner violence and obtaining as well as keeping employment (Browne, Salomon, & Bassuk, 1999). Anecdotal data gathered by the Taylor Institute described what impact partner violence had on a woman's ability to participate in a job training program or maintain work (Browne, Salomon, & Bassuk, 1999). Raphael (1999) outlined obstacles and barriers presented to women by their abusive partners when trying to achieve self-sufficiency. These barriers included, but were certainly not limited to, destruction of educational materials and showing up at the work site to harass them.

The data collected heightened concerns that the new welfare policy would place women in the dangerous situation of forcing them to stay with their abusive partners by not offering adequate supportive services to them. The Personal Responsibility and Work Opportunity Reconciliation Act addressed these concerns in two ways. The legislation stipulated that only 20% of a state's caseload qualified for exemption of time limits and its definition of hardship was battery and extreme cruelty (Browne, Salomon, & Bassuk, 1999). The Family Violence Option (FVO) "provided the states an opportunity to require certain standards and procedures, including screening welfare recipients for current danger from a violent intimate; referral to counseling and support services; and exemptions of requirements such as time limits, residency, child support enforcement, and family cap provisions" when a participant was in a dangerous situation and her safety would be compromised and the victim was being unfairly punished (Institute for Women's Policy Research, 1997, as stated in Browne, Salomon, & Bassuk, 1999).

With the enactment of the Family Violence Option legislation, the Department of Health and Human Services (DHHS) had to deal with three issues. The first one was the states' preoccupation with the idea that if too many women asked for the domestic violence waivers for work requirements, states would fail to meet their requirement and would ultimately lose their federal funding. The DHHS clarified and specified that if a state were to fail to meet the required work participation due to domestic violence waivers they would not be penalized. The second issue was that under the PRWORA states could not provide more than 20% of their total caseload with a "hardship exemption." What the proponents of the Family Violence Option intended to do was to expand the 20% "hardship exemption" category for welfare recipients with other hardships. DHHS agreed that the 20% limit could be exceeded if it was exceeded due to domestic violence waivers. The third major issue was the time limit for the Family Violence Option. The proposed legislation emphasized that the FVO waivers should not exceed 6 months (Raphael, 1999).

For such legislation to be successful there needs to be adequate screening and referral services by the staff in the welfare offices and employment training programs. Raphael (1999) assessed the Family Violence Option and its implementation in all 50 states, Puerto Rico, and in the District of Columbia. In all but 11 states, the time clock keeps ticking for victims of domestic violence and the time can only be extended if domestic violence is still a barrier to achieving or maintaining employment. The individual TANF worker is in the position to approve a temporary waiver for a TANF participant in all but a few states. The problem is that many of these workers were originally trained to screen for eligibility and need of job training and childcare. Now workers are being asked to assess for domestic violence also. The majority of states (35) are implementing a special method of assessment for identifying domestic violence. Only a few states (9) provided any type of information to recipients informing them about the advantages of disclosing to their workers if they were in a domestic violence situation. None of the states follow up with specific questions about domestic violence. In this study, one state's domestic violence coalition reported an inconsistency of information given to recipients and a lack of knowledge of policy in some of their local offices. This raises questions regarding the training that workers are receiving (Raphael, 1999).

SUBSTANCE ABUSE TREATMENT SERVICES/ MENTAL HEALTH SERVICES

The Department of Health and Human Services states that anywhere from 6 to 37% of welfare recipients have a substance abuse problem. Substance abuse has proven to pose a problem in moving recipients of welfare off public assistance and into work. In the area of substance abuse little research has concentrated on the evaluation of implementation of supportive services that would aid women moving from welfare to work. Due to the changing welfare system these issues have become increasingly important, particularly for drug-abusing women (Metsch, McCoy,

Miller, McAnany, & Pereyra, 1999). This issue is important because substance abuse, as well as domestic violence and mental health issues, acts as a barrier for women seeking employment or trying to maintain their current employment. The PRWORA addresses the issue of substance abuse in two ways. First, "it prohibits states from providing financial aid or food stamps to persons convicted of drug-related felonies." The PRWORA does give states the option of modifying this requirement or not accepting it at all. Secondly, it allows states to administer drug tests to "participants and to penalize those that test positive" (P.L. 104-193, as stated in Metsch, McCoy, Miller, McAnany, & Pereyra, 1999).

Even before PRWORA was enacted, substance abuse had been identified as a problem and a barrier in gaining and maintaining employment. According to recent studies on substance abuse, "employment rates among substance abusers are substantially lower than employment rates of non-substance abusers." Welfare recipients with substance abuse problems are also less likely to hold steady, full-time employment (Metsch, McCoy, Miller, McAnany, & Pereyra, 1999). Women with substance abuse problems are reported as having lower educational achievements, fewer job skills, and less job experience in comparison to men with substance abuse problems (Metsch, McCoy, Miller, McAnany, Pereyra, 1999). These findings coupled with time limits call for states and counties to address this issue.

Metsch, McCoy, Miller, McAnany, and Pereyra (1999) examined barriers and facilitators to gaining and maintaining employment among 100 low-income women. These women participated in a long-term residential substance abuse treatment program. The research established that there were several variables associated with the work status of the respondents. The first variable was the recipients having received some type of job training and having a higher education. The second variable was remaining "drug free." The third variable was successful completion of the Village (substance abuse treatment) program. The fourth variable was close relationships with friends. These respondents were more likely to be employed. An interesting observation that the authors made is that a close relationship with family members was not related to work status.

SUPPORTIVE SERVICES AND CALIFORNIA WELFARE POLICY

California established the California Work Opportunity and Responsibility to Kids Program or CalWORKS in response to the enactment of

TANF. CalWORKS is intended to move welfare recipients into jobs. The federal policy offered states the option of adopting the Family Violence Option, which mandates workers to screen for domestic violence and make the appropriate referrals. Another stipulation of the legislation is a waiver from time limits for domestic violence victims. This allows the worker to waive the victim's work requirement for up to 6 months without the states being sanctioned. California is one of the states that opted to accept this legislation. State legislation required individual counties to set up screening and referrals to supportive services to better serve the participants' needs. In most counties, supportive services are being offered only to those recipients NOT exempt from work requirements. However, Los Angeles County declared exempt adults eligible for county-funded domestic violence services (California Institute for Mental Health, 2000).

This policy has made the focus for CalWORKS caseworkers one of screening for domestic violence, drug and alcohol treatment, and mental health services. The priority is not on helping. Rather, this screening is to provide referrals to services, with the priority on getting participants off welfare and in the paid labor force and meeting the mandated time limits. Before the change in policy, workers were trained for eligibility and employment finding only. Due to the change in policy, CalWORKS caseworkers now have the power to sanction a participant for not meeting work requirements or waive a participant's work requirements. This added responsibility makes worker training vital because workers are now responsible for implementing this new policy. They must help recipients understand the policy so they can follow through on obtaining needed services. At the same time, workers must meet federal mandates of getting women off the welfare rolls and into employment or marriage to prevent federal funding cuts. Since evaluation of caseworkers' ability to do this difficult job is scarce, this research focuses on the evaluation of implementation of the supportive services policy by talking to participants and listening to how they learned about these services from the workers. In this study, we asked participants if and how CalWORKS offices and caseworkers are informing participants about services for domestic violence, substance abuse, and mental health services as well as ways to improve this process for the benefit of the participants.

METHODOLOGY

The researchers conducted five focus groups throughout Los Angeles County, one in the city of Los Angeles and four in the San Fernando Valley (Glendale, Northridge, and Van Nuys). Access was successful at four different agencies–a community advocacy and alcohol prevention agency, a social service agency, a domestic violence program, and a mental health center.[1] One focus group was held at each agency with the exception of the domestic violence program, where two focus groups were held. Although most of the participants were receiving mainly domestic violence services, a few were receiving mental health services, a few only drug and alcohol services, and a few received a combination of all three types of services. Our primary purpose was to explore how participants had learned about the services from their CalWORKS' caseworkers. A secondary concern was to ask for suggestions on how this information on the supportive service process could be improved.

Three of the focus groups consisted of women who met on a regular basis. One group met monthly for advocacy purposes at an agency to help women stay drug free, and the other two regular groups met weekly for support at a local domestic violence shelter (one Spanish-speaking and one English-speaking group). The other two focus groups were held with participants who came together only for the interview–one at a local mental health agency and one at a local social service agency with a long-term housing program.

SAMPLE

Almost two-thirds (19) of the 30 adult participants self-identified their race/ethnicity as Latina/o American/Hispana/o/ic, followed by White/Caucasian (6), Black/African-American (4), and White and Indian (1). In line with national statistics showing that over 95% of adult participants are female, 29 of the 30 participants were female. At the participants' request/need, Spanish translation was provided for one group, three groups were held in English only, and one group was held in Spanish only. The median (and mean) age was 34 and the age range was 21 to 50. The median number of months on AFDC/TANF was 24, with a range of 3 months to 9 years. The median number of children was 2.5, with a range of 1 to 8 children. About two-thirds (19) of the participants had high school degrees or GEDs and nearly one-third (9) were currently working.

FINDINGS

When asked how they learned about supportive services, the participants explained that their CalWORKS caseworkers provided insufficient information at best and discouraged them from obtaining services at worst. In several instances, participants were informed of supportive services by other sources, oftentimes after their caseworkers had either ignored or denied the participant's request for help. In a few instances, the worker was very helpful in providing information about supportive services.

Insufficient and Insensitive Information from CalWORKS Caseworkers

When participants answered "yes" to the application's close-ended question asking if there was a need for domestic violence, drug and alcohol treatment, or mental health counseling, caseworkers would sometimes ignore this information.

> In my case, I needed help two years ago. I filed papers and I remember that there's a form where they ask you [about domestic violence] and I signed and dated it and gave it to my worker and she gave it back and said, "I don't need that." She gave it back in a big protest and in a month they declined my application and so I reapplied because people that I knew told me I had to because I had no other choice and so I did it again and this time they did accept it [the application], but the paper, I signed it again and again they gave it back. I still have it at home.

In some cases, they would be referred to a domestic violence caseworker and still obtain no help.

> So I went there and the form that I had to fill out, I put that I was a domestic violence client. They referred me to a domestic [violence] person that [was] supposed to help you know just fill out the papers. She took proof of everything and that was it. She didn't say anything else. I was kind of shocked because I was expecting you know for her to explain this is what you would be entitled to if you did this or not. But she didn't say nothing, she was just doing her job.

One woman who was turned away without obtaining the help she sought went back into denial about her domestic abuse.

> Well, I originally went to apply like in 1999, a year after I was in domestic violence. At the time, I didn't know it was domestic violence situation. But the legal papers were there, the restraining [order], all that stuff was there. So when I went to apply I remember

they gave me a whole bunch of papers and I filled them out. They gave me ten days, a week or so, to go back. I went back and I remember . . . I actually took the legal papers. I remember the worker, I gave her the whole bunch of papers and then she just looked at me then. The ones she need, she put on the side; the ones she return to me, she put them on the other. Then I found the one that had the question of domestic violence, she put [it] on the side, she was going to return to me. She gave it back to me and I told her, "Don't you need this?" "Oh, no, we don't need that." So she put it aside.

She later explained that this was her third time applying; that the same thing had happened the first two times and that caused her to deny her abuse. When they gave the paperwork back to her the second time, she explained her thoughts:

I stop and I said, "Well, I guess I wasn't in a domestic violence situation. I guess I am wrong and I started feeling guilty. And actually it took more than a year for me to get convinced by my friend and my parents to see my situation . . . they actually gave me I think an affidavit where I had to write. They told me to fill out and explain what had happened with my batterer. He tried to take my kids and you know he was pretty violent. I find it in everything [referring to her CalWORKS paperwork] even they filed it, everything, they filed it and I [still] didn't get help.

Other clients reported active discouragement and rudeness when they reported their need for domestic violence services. Caseworkers rejected the women's active requests for help.

I told her that I need to get out of the home. The guy was battering me. The worker told me: "Well, why don't you stay with your baby's daddy?" Look, I'm calling because of my baby's daddy. The worker responded: "You don't have to catch an attitude."

I don't know if I did then or not [check the box stating she needed help with domestic violence]. But when I recertified this past year in September, I did. I wrote down that I was and the worker at the time, she said, "Are you sure you want to write this?" Like yea. Because she was trying to talk me out of it and you I know I am like yea. She said that means you are going to have a different worker. I am thinking that it doesn't matter.

Help from Advocates Other than CalWORKS Caseworkers

Participants often learned of their right to supportive services from other sources, namely legal and social service advocates and health care providers. Several of the women learned about their right to CalWORKS supportive services from domestic violence shelter staff and/or program staff, lawyers at court or from Legal Aid, child protective service workers, court social workers, doctors, and television programs. Sometimes they learned about services from flyers and brochures or from their GAIN (California's welfare-to-work job training program) worker. All of these providers served as advocates for the clients with the welfare worker. In several incidents, the participants were still not given help from their caseworker until they asserted their right to see the caseworker's supervisor.

In the two situations explained in the previous section, where the women's requests for help were ignored, they were referred to GAIN and it was here that they were finally helped.

> ... and then after 5 months, they call me from GAIN and scheduled an appointment and so I go. They started telling me for a whole month that I needed to find a job. At the moment that I went I was going through a difficult time, an emotional time, and I broke down in her office and she told me to hold on that she knew of someone and so she called here [the domestic violence center].
>
> I found out two months later through the mail that I did qualify for aid and then four months later my GAIN worker called. I was going though a really, really hard situation still. I just broke down in one of her appointments at the GAIN. She really wanted me to start working. I told her that I really needed some kind of counseling and guidance or I'd have a nervous breakdown. I didn't know what to do and she told me hold on. She turned her head and she looked for a number and she called here [to the domestic violence program]. She set up an appointment with the person that was working here at the time. It was a Friday; I came down and from then on I come in here.

However, in most instances, it was professionals outside of the welfare system that informed women about their right to supportive services. Many participants found out about services at the domestic violence shelters where the staff referred them back to the welfare office so they could obtain referrals to domestic violence programs. Domestic violence program advocates then helped participants work with their CalWORKS caseworker to obtain benefits, prevent sanctions (being cut off from benefits due to alleged lack of follow through), and obtain appropriate waivers from finding employment or reaching their welfare-receipt time limits.

Other professionals also played an active role in informing women about supportive services.

> I found out about help because of my lawyer from Legal Aid. She referred me here (to the alcohol and drug abuse treatment agency) and she told me I could receive more aid from welfare because I was a victim of domestic violence.

This woman was initially denied aid because she was an immigrant without legal documentation. The worker was "very rude," telling her the papers she brought from immigration "weren't worth anything" and that they "didn't mean anything." The worker went on to say she "had no aid to give her." The participant obtained a letter from the Legal Aid lawyer and it was then that the welfare worker "took me seriously."

Another participant explained that her doctor informed her about mental health support services. She was with the GAIN program at the time.

> I learned from a regular doctor because I had problems. I was a young mom; I have not finished high school . . . my regular doctor figured out that I wasn't well [she was diagnosed with clinical depression] and that I had to have a therapist . . . I said well how do I do this? He said you go and you have to get the papers from your GAIN worker and fill them out.

In several instances, CalWORKS caseworkers would help participants only after the participants demanded to see their supervisor. One woman's story illustrates this situation in a most dramatic way, one that illustrates further abuse by the worker. After she asked for services, the worker "rocked in his chair and said 'Well, I'm not going to give you those services.'" She continued:

> Maybe you are not understanding me or I may not be explaining myself but I am a domestic violence victim and from what I under-

stand from my friends, I know there is this, this, and that. He said, "I already told you NO."

Their conversation continued in the same vein until she said "Oh, so you want to control ME." He said, "Yes."

> I told him [if I wanted] to be controlled, I would have stayed with my abuser. I had to make a scene there. The supervisor came and everything and I told her I don't want this type of man as my worker.

Frequently, women resolved their lack of information or poor treatment from caseworkers by asking and sometimes demanding to see the supervisor. The woman mentioned earlier, whose worker told her to stay with the father, is a typical example. She took action by going to the supervisor.

> So I went to the supervisor and the supervisor assisted me and got this lady off my case. I mean domestic violence is nothing to play with and she took it as something of a joke I guess. You know, I also got a lot of help through the county and then I didn't get a lot of help through the county.

Good Caseworkers

In a few cases, clients reported that their workers were very helpful. These workers referred participants directly to providers and quickly returned calls. One woman explained that at the Long Beach office, "When it comes down to domestic violence, they are right there. They do assist you in different things that you need. . . . They put you in shelters where if your abuser is controlling, they put [you] in a hide-away shelter."

Participants expressed appreciation for competent and compassionate workers. One woman gives an example of a good worker who took time to empathize with her situation:

> And as far as the social workers, the one that I spoke to today, Mr. I can't say his name. He was very compassionate and understanding; he wasn't pretending. He told me he would call me back and he did. And, um, I respect and appreciated that because he did show some concern for my situation. And he also gave me a pointer that he wasn't

supposed to or probably was off the record. But he said he had a handicapped child and he understood.

She went on to explain how she appreciated another worker who clearly explained her options to her. Another participant agreed that she had a worker who she liked for the same reason.

> [H]e did research prior to giving me an answer. He said, let me call you back and see what I can find out for you instead of saying, "Well, no the guidelines say this, and this is how it goes." You know, he had enough courtesy and compassion to see what other options I had, which was appreciated by me because he showed me some concern.

Fear and Distrust of Caseworkers and the System in General

Participants expressed fear and distrust of asking for help from the CalWORKS caseworker. There fears centered around being treated poorly because of the stigma associated with mental illness, drug and alcohol abuse, and domestic violence, or losing their children because they would be reported to child protective services. One Spanish-speaking participant explained that the caseworker did ask her, "Are you in a domestic violence situation? Are you on drugs/alcohol?" She said she was in a domestic violence situation and they asked her, do you want help/services, and she said she didn't want any. Later she explained that she felt fear that if she said yes, she would lose her children. She felt "more like I have to do it on my own and figure out my own solution because I don't feel like they are gonna help me." Another woman expressed her fears about stigma and losing her children. As she talked, all of the focus group members strongly expressed their agreement with her thoughts both by saying yes and nodding their heads vehemently. She began working six years ago at $5.35 an hour and had advanced to $10 an hour and described her anger at being refused help from CalWORKS in the following manner.

> ... then the terrorist strike came and I got injured and they told me, 'cause like I said my daughter was on SSI, that I made too much money. And as far as those drug programs and mental health, you know I don't trust the system because they say they want to help but a lot of times they just want to take your kids away from you. And I had alcohol problems; I was an alcoholic and I still consider myself an alcoholic and a recovering addict. But I went to AA my-

> self and to church and um, by the mercy of God, was able to obtain and maintain some sort of sobriety. But I would not trust them, if I went to them; they said if you have CalWORKS, you can go to the Tarzana treatment center. And I said, "Like hell." I'm sure then I'll be on the books as an alcoholic or an addict and they'll follow me around and they'll make sure that if I ever make a mistake, they'll take my kids. The system, you can't trust 'em like that; they mean well but then again some of them don't.

The fear of child protective services existed in spite of the fact that child protective service involvement also helped some clients obtain fair treatment from the CalWORKS caseworker. For example, a child protective services worker referred one woman to parenting classes. Her CalWORKS caseworker did not refer her to any domestic violence programs even though she informed the worker she was a victim of domestic violence.

> ... my ex-husband filed a report claiming I abuse my kids. The social worker came, reviewed my kids and the case and didn't find anything. He sent me to parenting classes to do 12 sessions but I stayed there. I have two years there now. So there in the parenting classes I spoke with the person giving the classes and told them what was going on. So he said coincidentally last week someone came from another agency to explain their program. It had been [a well-respected domestic violence program]. ... They gave me the number ... and I took action. But my welfare worker would only tell ... me, "You have to go to therapy, you have to go to counseling" ... she never told me where to go.

Less-specific fears were also expressed: fear of losing aid when that aid was desperately needed, fear of caseworkers' yelling which triggers memories of abuse, and general fear and distrust of the welfare system, especially when dealing with immigration issues (see earlier quote). One woman explained how her aid had been incorrectly taken away from her and only after the domestic violence program staff person intervened and advocated on her behalf did a supervisor step in and reinstate her benefits. She summarized her experience by explaining how she felt while dealing with several caseworkers that continually denied her benefits.

> That was my experience with welfare. But many times they are not with us. They see us like a case number. Sometimes, for example, as

victims of domestic violence, we are very sensitive and of course if they are going to tell us, "I don't care about your case" (she yelled this sentence), we are going to get scared and many times they trigger trauma from our abuse. They are not, they don't have feelings. They are cold. They are despotic.

Suggestions to Improve the Information Given by Caseworkers

All participants suggested that the caseworkers be more sensitive to their situations. For some that meant being aware of the general reason they are there: to apply for aid because they are in a financial crisis. For others, that meant being aware of the compassion and calm way survivors of trauma need to be treated. One woman's experience typifies how fear and anger can trigger participants to respond in kind.

> I had the experience once at welfare that the lady cancelled my aid and I was calling her to give her my documents and she was talking to me very aggressively. Because she was doing this, I got nervous and started crying and I started shouting out of anger. So she told me, "You know what I'm not going to talk to you." She turned around and walked away. So I got very angry and I said, "Oh, no, this is not going to stay like this." So I went to the receptionist and told him I needed to talk to someone because the worker did this and this and she was screaming. He was very good. He said (in a whisper), "You know what, talk to the deputy."

After creating a commotion and being approached by a guard, she did get the attention of the deputy who took her aside, listened to her story, brought the worker in, made the worker apologize to the participant, and provided her with the proposed assistance.

Other suggestions included training caseworkers to be capable and conscious of the needs of domestic violence survivors:

> The welfare workers don't know. They don't know how to treat domestic violence. If they trained a few people to deal with people that are there for domestic violence, they would understand and not try to intimidate people and threaten them with, "I'm going to close your case."

Two specific suggestions were made for changes in the system. The first was the use of a better questioning system. Instead of just asking the one closed-ended question, one woman suggested that a series of questions would be more sensitive and more informative.

> You know I didn't really realize how bad things are and how abused I was until I went through like the checklist here [at the domestic violence program] and I was like, oh my goodness oh my goodness. Because most people think hitting, ending up in the hospital [is the only indicator of domestic abuse]. What I was thinking while you were speaking maybe a suggestion would be instead of just one little sentence, are you domestically, have you been abused? Some women don't even really realize what that means. So how about a little yes and no question to even let the women even realize it. Obviously when someone hits you, you realize it, but yea the money abuse, the verbal abuse, the emotional abuse, I think it takes awhile to sink in.

Along with being treated with understanding, "compassion, empathy, and sympathy," participants want to be accurately informed about the services available to them and then given phone numbers and referrals. One woman said she was told that the county could help her with her first and last month's rent for an apartment so that she could move away from the abuser. She did not get this help, nor did she get an explanation of what the county could or could not do for her; instead, she was curtly referred to a shelter where she was told she had to pay to stay.

DISCUSSION: SUGGESTIONS FOR IMPROVING THE SUPPORTIVE SERVICE DELIVERY SYSTEM

Increase Attention on Caseworkers. Caseworkers are put in an extremely difficult situation. They are to assess for eligibility, implement a complicated policy, and do at least an initial screening for participants in need of domestic violence services, alcohol and drug abuse treatment, and mental health services. They are to carry out this task with limited training, low pay, large caseloads, and pressure from administrators to keep in mind the priority–reduce caseloads and push women into work in the paid labor force–to prevent federal funding cuts. They are working in an agency that has a history of abysmal treatment of its applicants. However, in spite of these difficult job tasks, participants clearly stated that some, albeit a minority of, caseworkers were helpful, compassionate, empathetic, and informative concerning supportive services. This information is important to keep in mind as we call for improvement in the system and training of caseworkers.

Caseworkers as a general rule need extensive training concerning supportive services' policy and how to deal with participants who are in very stressful situations. Participants made it very clear that most caseworkers lack knowledge of available resources and sensitivity to interviewing participants who have experienced trauma, violence, mental illness, and substance abuse while also facing conditions of severe poverty. Participants suggested that caseworkers need to understand the dynamics of dealing with women and trauma, particularly women who are living in or recently have lived in domestic violence situations. Most domestic violence programs provide training for their volunteer staff. It would be easy to incorporate some of this training into the caseworkers' training. Also, involving some of the identified "good" caseworkers in training programs would be beneficial for other workers and cost-effective for welfare agencies.

Participants made it clear that when they were able to talk to supervisors, they often got their needs met by the caseworkers. Supervisors need to become more actively involved in training and ongoing contact with workers. Supervisory support can help caseworkers implement their training and spot some problems for future training purposes. Ongoing supervisory support for caseworkers would also relieve participants of the stressful situation of having to demand to see the supervisor.

Improve the Presentation About Supportive Services in the Application Screening Question. What appears to be a simple, straightforward application question to initially screen for domestic violence, alcohol/drug abuse, and mental health issues is not adequate in this context. Sometimes, participants are non-responsive to this question due to fears of being poorly treated, losing custody of their children, and/or being stigmatized by the government. Other times, this question is simply unnecessary because many participants openly talk about their issues when they initially apply for welfare. This question needs to be revised so that it allows the applicant to see her situation with clarity (e.g., perhaps a simple series of questions to help her identify if she is indeed in need of further assessment).

When a participant does identify herself (either through a sensitive screening questionnaire or by self-identifying) in need of supportive services, it is vital that the caseworker have a safe, sensitive, and effective system for providing the participant with accurate, non-judgmental, and clear referrals. It is also imperative that the participant be given a chance to get help and know the consequences of what may come later should she choose not to act on the referrals. Any threat of sanctions or negative consequences at this time is inappropriate and a set-up for failure. Waivers should be fully explained and granted in the case of domestic violence, especially waivers for women who are immigrants. Supervisors must support the caseworkers in carrying out these actions with participants. Caseworkers must receive adequate information in all of these policy implementation issues as well as an opportunity to role play these situations before they actually deal directly with participants.

Provide for an Assessment System that Actively Involves Advocates. Participants made it very clear that the advocates either from the GAIN side of the welfare program or from professionals outside of the welfare office (e.g., teachers, lawyers, agency workers, and court social workers) are key players in learning about supportive services and welfare policy. These advocates need to be more actively incorporated into the training and education of the caseworkers. Such involvement would also provide an opportunity for caseworkers to obtain information on how to allay participants' fears that they will have their children taken away from them if they are honest with the caseworkers. At the very least, assessing the need for reporting the family to Child Protective Services or not could be left up to the advocates, instead of the CalWORKS caseworkers.

CONCLUSION

This paper offers information directly from welfare participants that can be used to begin to further evaluate and improve the implementation of the new welfare policy concerning informing clients about supportive services, namely domestic violence, substance abuse, and mental health services. The women we talked to during these focus groups were clearly struggling to improve their lives and the lives of their children under the dire circumstances of poverty and domestic violence, alcohol and drug addiction, mental illness, or a combination of all of these factors. They were not only willing to talk to us about their experiences in learning about these supportive services from their welfare caseworkers but they were willing to share their stories and ideas with us. They did this in spite of the fact that it was painful for them.

In a system with a policy that is lengthy and complicated as well as hidden from the daily lives of most of us, participants seem to be the best informants about how the policy is implemented. Certainly, participants who are actively trying to change their lives by participating in support groups and simultaneously maintaining their benefits through public assistance are a valuable resource for understanding how we can improve the welfare system. As one of our participants said, "We are doing this because we do want to work; we want to value ourselves. We want to get our kids a different life. We need people trained . . . that understand."

REFERENCES

Abramovitz, M. (1988). *Regulating the lives of women: Social welfare policy from colonial times to the present.* (Chapter 10). Boston: South End Press.

Browne, A., Salomon, A., & Bassuk, S. S. (1999). The impact of recent partner violence on poor women's capacity to maintain work. *Violence Against Women,* 5(4), 393-426.

Brush, L. (1999). Woman battering and welfare reform: The view from a welfare-to-work program. *Journal of Sociology and Social Welfare,* 264(3), 49-60.

California Institute for Mental Health (along with Children and Family Futures and Family Violence Prevention Fund). (2000, April). The CalWORKS project: Six county case study–Alameda, Kern, Los Angeles, Monterey, Shasta, Stanislaus project report. Sacramento, CA, pp. 1-9 (Introduction). *http://www.cimh.org*

Cancian, M., & Meyer, D. R. (2000). Work after Welfare: Women's Work Effort, Occupation, and Economic Well-Being. *Social Work Research,* 24(2), 69-86.

Danziger, S., Corcoran, M., Danziger, S., & Heflin, C. M. (2000). Work, Income, and Material Hardship after Welfare Reform. *Journal of Consumer Affairs,* 34(1), 6-30.

Harrington, M. (1962). *The other America: Poverty in the United States.* New York: Macmillan Co.

Jimenez, M. A. (1999). A Feminist Analysis of Welfare Reform: The Personal Responsibility Act of 1996. *Affilia,* 144(3), 278-293.

Metsch, L.R., McCoy, C.B., Miller, M., McAnany, H., & Pereyra, M. (1999). Moving substance abusing women from welfare to work. *Journal of Public Health Policy,* 20(1), 36-51.

Meyers, M.K., Han, W., Waldfogel, J., & Garfinkel, I. (2001). Child care in the wake of welfare reform: The impact of government subsidies on the economic well-being of single mother families. *Social Service Review,* 75(1), 29-59.

O'Campo, P., & Rojas-Smith, L. (1998). Welfare reform and women's health: Review of the literature and implications for state policy. *Journal of Public Health Policy,* 19(4), 420-443.

Raphael, J. (1999). The family violence option : An early assessment. *Violence Against Women,* 5(4), 449-466.

Rose, N. E. (2000). Scapegoating Poor Women: An Analysis of Welfare Reform. *Journal of Economic Issues,* 34(1), 143-157.

Swigonski, M. E. (1996). Women, Poverty, and Welfare Reform: A Challenge to Social Workers. *Journal of Women and Social Work,* 11(1), 95-110.

Woolis, D.D. (1998). Family Works: Substance Abuse Treatment and Welfare Reform. *Public Welfare,* 56(1), 24-31.

Making Experience Count in Policy Creation: Lessons from Appalachian Kentucky

Christiana Miewald

SUMMARY. An emphasis on work as the solution to poverty–"work first"–has become the model for public assistance policy since 1996. For poor communities, however, work alone will not solve issues of poverty. In Appalachian Kentucky low-income parents need access to education in order to find living wage employment. Through the strategic use of media and the creation of legislation, activists are able to challenge work first policies and help to craft programs that meet local needs. This paper examines the process by which myths about welfare, work and responsibility are inscribed into policy and discusses efforts by low-income parents and welfare rights advocates to transform those policies. It concludes by arguing that to address the issues of poverty, public assistance policy must take into account the lived experience of low-income parents. *[Article copies available for a fee from The Haworth Document Delivery Service:*

Christiana Miewald has a PhD in anthropology from the University of Kentucky and is a visiting scholar in the geography department at the Ohio State University.

Address correspondence to: Christiana Miewald, PhD, Department of Geography, 1036 Derby Hall, The Ohio State University, Columbus, OH 43210-1361.

The author would like to thank the generous support of those individuals who facilitated this research, including members of the Kentucky Welfare Reform Coalition, Appalshop, Kentuckians for the Commonwealth and Kentucky Youth Advocates.

This research was supported by a National Science Foundation Dissertation Improvement Grant (9615837).

[Haworth co-indexing entry note]: "Making Experience Count in Policy Creation: Lessons from Appalachian Kentucky." Miewald, Christiana. Co-published simultaneously in *Journal of Poverty* (The Haworth Press, Inc.) Vol. 7, No. 1/2, 2003, pp. 163-181; and: *Rediscovering the Other America: The Continuing Crisis of Poverty and Inequality in the United States* (ed: Keith M. Kilty, and Elizabeth A. Segal) The Haworth Press, Inc., 2003, pp. 163-181. Single or multiple copies of this article are available for a fee from The Haworth Document Delivery Service [1-800-HAWORTH, 9:00 a.m. - 5:00 p.m. (EST). E-mail address: docdelivery@haworthpress.com].

© 2003 by The Haworth Press, Inc. All rights reserved.

1-800-HAWORTH. E-mail address: <docdelivery@haworthpress.com> Website: <http://www.HaworthPress.com> © 2003 by The Haworth Press, Inc. All rights reserved.]

KEYWORDS. Political activism, Appalachia, welfare reform

INTRODUCTION

This paper examines efforts by parents, grassroots activists and state-wide organizations to reconfigure the Kentucky Transitional Assistance Program through a multi-scale analysis of policy and agency. I begin by examining how myths about welfare, work and responsibility are currently inscribed into policy (Thomas, 1997). Here, I look at two basic trends in federal and state welfare policies–an emphasis on work as the solution to poverty and a reliance on "local solutions" in order to move recipients from "welfare to work." I then examine how these trends have been implemented at the state level within the Kentucky Transitional Assistance Program or K-TAP. It is at the level of the state where contradictions often emerge between federal rhetoric and local economic and social realities. Finally, I describe the process by which federal welfare rhetoric and state policies are contested by groups in Appalachian Kentucky through the strategic use of media, organizing and the creation of legislation. Using these examples, I explore the ways in which local experience can be used to challenge the welfare myths and how organizations are creating spaces at the local and state levels to assert their own visions of welfare.

As I inquire into the connections between mythmaking, policymaking and local experience, I ask whether it is possible, in this age of governmental devolution, for local knowledge to influence public policy at higher levels of power. This issue is addressed with an ethnographic attention to the lived experience of public assistance in Appalachian Kentucky as well as a concern for how that lived experience might be most effectively translated into policy. Specifically, I employ three lenses through which to view recent changes to welfare policy–(1) Transcripts from the congressional debate on welfare reform in 1995 and 1996 which highlight the national-level rhetoric of work-first and devolution, (2) Participant observation at the state level where Kentucky welfare policy is constructed and contested and (3) An ethnographic examination of representational and policy strategies emerging from local communities in Appalachian Kentucky. Appalachia, like other economically distressed regions, is particularly vulnerable to the negative effects of current welfare policy because of its long-standing poverty, lack of job opportunities and economic reliance on transfer payments. Yet because of these conditions, it is where Kentucky's welfare policies are most often subject to critique.

The emphasis on 'work-first' at the federal and state levels can result in a mismatch between policy and local conditions–especially in economically marginalized regions such as the Mississippi Delta, Native American reservations and Appalachia (Harvey et al., 2002). While states are delegated the responsibility of creating welfare programs that meet local conditions and needs, states must also enforce work requirements, meet federal participation rates and adhere to federal definitions of work (Mink, 1998, p. 65). In the case of Appalachian Kentucky, "work-first" policies do not meet local labor market conditions, nor do they address the need for education and training. At the same time, devolution of welfare planning has opened up spaces for political action–a possibility for the emergence of progressive policies from contradictions betwen state policy and local conditions. The question is whether these challenges to the federal emphasis on work can bubble up from the local scale to influence state and federal policy.

Within the current welfare debate, places with high poverty are once again framed as culturally and morally deviant. This, in turn, acts as a rationalizing metaphor to galvanize public support for the withdrawal of the social safety net (Francis-Okongwu, 1995). Perhaps most problematic is the notion that single parenthood, drug use and crime are due to a "culture of poverty" or, more recently, a "culture of welfare." This explanation for poverty is based on the notion that it is caused by individual or cultural dysfunction, rather than structural inequalities (Gilbert, 1997; Schram, 2000; Seccombe et al., 1999).

Thus, in the paper, I argue that in order to challenge dominant representations of welfare and to facilitate political action, there is a need to promote and disseminate information that reflects the realities of welfare policies for individuals, families and communities. One strategy is to translate lived experience about welfare into direct challenges of policy. Such a strategy, which is being employed by a coalition of progressive organizations in Kentucky, actively contests the myths upon which current welfare policy is constructed and provides an avenue for alternatives to the work-first approach.

POVERTY MYTHS AND PUBLIC POLICY

In the first section of this paper, I investigate the relationships between mythmaking and policymaking within the recent reconfiguration of the

American welfare system, otherwise known as welfare reform. I begin with the premise that the power to represent is the power to establish what stands for legitimate knowledge. What counts as knowledge and how it is circulated and controlled through discourse is central to the creation and implementation of public policy. While the production of discourses surrounding welfare has been largely controlled by federal rhetoric, devolution provides opportunities for representational strategies aimed at countering the dominant mythology. Thus, as welfare is reconfigured within the framework of the Personal Responsibility and Work Opportunity Reconciliation Act, what is emerging at the local level are confrontations over who has the power to articulate the lived experience of welfare within the public policy arena.

Welfare policy, in the words of Nancy Fraser (1990, p. 203) has become "a site of struggle where groups with unequal discursive (and nondiscursive) resources compete to establish as hegemonic their respective interpretations of legitimate social needs." To date, the power to represent the "facts" of welfare has been dominated by neoconservative politicians and mainstream media. Those directly affected by changes in public assistance are not involved in the decision-making process, nor are there many avenues through which to tell their side of the story.

Within the debate that surrounded the passage of the Personal Responsibility and Work Opportunity Reconciliation Act, myths were employed to depict the failure of federal welfare programs and the cultural "pathologies" that these programs were said to cause. In the mythology of welfare, the poor are presented as culturally different from the majority, a 'deviant' subculture or an 'underclass' prone to illegitimacy, crime and debasement of the community (Cerullo and Erlien, 1996). The circulation and acceptance of welfare myths is noted by Albelda and Tilly (1996, p. 79) who comment, "Hating poor women for being poor is all the rage. Radio talk show hosts, conservative think tanks and many elected officials bash poor single mothers for being too 'lazy,' too 'dependent' and too fertile."

But why have myths become so pervasive in the national welfare debate? Lawmakers circulate myths because they give their arguments the power of popular opinion and because, as members of society, legislators are likely to believe them (Thomas, 1997). For policymakers, welfare myths provide powerful rhetorical tools for managing public opinion and framing the debate. For those in political and economic power, controlling how welfare is represented and understood within the public sphere is a vital component to ensuring that policies are not contested. Piven and Cloward (1997) observe that voter preferences in most policy areas are ambiguous and shifting, especially for issues where people have little direct knowledge. Residential apartheid in urban areas and the isolation of poor rural communities means that much of suburban America learns about welfare through the mainstream media, where stereotypical portrayals reinforce the belief that public assistance is the cause of economic and social ills. This lack of public knowledge about the realities of living on welfare, combined with a general antipathy toward the poor, are often used by politicians to support punitive social policies (Flanders 1996).

But myths are not simply symbolic constructs or rhetorical devices; they often have the power to influence both political action and material circumstances. According to Andrew Maxwell (1996), myths "constitute an element in the maintenance of a societal ideology which serves to rationalize, and thus undergird, the objective process of capital accumulation and related immiseration." For Maxwell, shifts in capital accumulation strategies since the 1970s have contributed to the transformation from public assistance to the "correctional-industrial complex" as a means of containing and disciplining surplus labor. Thus, workfare or "work-first" policies may be viewed as part of a post-Fordist accumulation strategy that relies on flexibility of production and labor practices. Flexibility is also central to the devolution of responsibility for public assistance programs, which, in turn, is part of a larger "hollowing out" of the nation-state (Peck, 1998). States and localities can now exert a more direct and specialized influence on public assistance programs. Among the trends associated with workfare strategies are the imposition of stringent work requirements, the application of different forms of compulsion to participate in make-work schemes or employment, heightened surveillance of individuals, and demonizing of welfare recipients by political elites—or mythmaking. Representative Clay Shaw Jr. of Florida, for example, plays upon racialized images of an urban underclass, mired in the culture of poverty, that threatens the middle class, both morally and physically:

> We all know the list of horrors: Crack babies who start out life from the first day with two strikes against them. The plague of illegitimacy in our inner cities. . . . Children giving birth to children who, we know, will be dramatically more susceptible to low birth weight, disease, physical abuse and drug addiction. An epidemic of violence the likes of which this country has never seen before. If some enemy of our country wanted to undermine the fabric of American society, it could not inflict anything upon us worse than the welfare system we have inflicted on ourselves. (Shaw, 1996)

In this portrayal, drug addiction, violence and illegitimacy are social diseases caused by the welfare system, which discourages work, penalizes marriage, and destroys personal responsibility and self-worth. The post-industrial image of dependency–the black, unwed, welfare-dependent mother– is, according to Fraser and Gordon (1996, p. 255), "a powerful ideological stereotype that simultaneously organizes diffuse cultural anxieties and dissimulates their social bases." Structural causes of poverty such as the lack of living-wage jobs and the effect of economic restructuring are simply not part of the problem.

Mythmaking has not only created an image of welfare programs and their effects but also provides the ideological basis of policymaking. In the following testimony, Senator Jon Kyl of Arizona presents us with what he see as the immutable facts of welfare–that "nonwork" and illegitimacy are key underlying causes of the "welfare crisis." The only remedy for this crisis is work and it is the state's responsibility to determine how best to get recipients into the waged labor market. Quoting Senator Kyl,

> Let us deal with the facts: To escape poverty and get off welfare, able-bodied individuals must enter and stay in the workforce. Once again: the Federal solution has been a failure. States can probably do better. States should be given the flexibility to determine how they will increase the number of welfare recipients engaged in work–and I mean *real* work. A number of studies . . . indicate that getting a welfare recipient into work is more likely than any other factor–more than training or education–to result in the recipient leaving welfare for good. (Kyl, 1995)

Within this mythic system, poverty is caused by a failure to work and therefore formerly irresponsible recipients must be made to work in order to get themselves out of poverty. Federal work requirements, time limits on benefits, sanctions for noncompliance, and the elimination of assistance for those deemed socially unworthy, such as immigrants and convicted drug felons, are policies directed toward disciplining the individual, rather than addressing social inequality.

The new responsibility for welfare also presents state governments with new challenges for finding local solutions within the framework of moving people from welfare to work. In areas with constricted labor markets or other barriers to employment, this means that states would be forced either to rectify employment and service inequalities or to become increasingly punitive in their efforts to ensure they meet federal participation rates.

K-TAP: KENTUCKY'S TANF PROGRAM

It is at the state level where federal mandates for "work-first" may conflict with the character of local economic and social geographies. The Kentucky Transitional Assistance Program, or K-TAP, reflects the national concern for "work-first" and relies on rhetoric of "local solutions" to the welfare policy. As mentioned above, devolution and work-first may be thought of as interrelated policies aimed at allowing localities greater flexibility in incorporating recipients into the waged labor market. Following the federal trend toward devolution, Kentucky has also emphasized the discovery of "creative" and "innovative" responses to persistent poverty in Appalachian Kentucky through local citizen involvement in policy formation.

How much flexibility and innovation are allowed within the planning process, however, has been dictated by federal definitions of work and the necessity for states to meet participation rates. As Peck (1998, p. 66) notes, even early experimentation with state and local welfare programs was predetermined by parameters set at the federal level–"demonstrations would seek generally low-cost ways of enforcing work, drawing on different combinations of job search and community service requirements."

Within state-sponsored forums, problems that are allowed to be addressed locally are only those related to social service provision and to programs aimed at making recipients "work ready." Calls to stop the timeclock, eliminate work requirements for students, or to provide more educational opportunities and living-wage jobs are met with resistance by state agents who cite budgetary constraints and pressure to comply with federal regulations. K-TAP, according to officials, is not an anti-poverty program nor is it an education program. Rather, it follows federal policy in focusing on moving recipients from welfare to work. One member of a Kentucky welfare advocacy coalition noted that while some members of state government have adopted a work-first, no excuses mentality,

> Federal law has really powerful incentives on states in the fact that it's very limited in how [education] counts toward your participation. And states may be acting rationally in response to that incentive. I think it's the wrong incentive though. That's how it looks from the state level. It's a completely mixed message. You would think that a block grant, by its very nature, involves a great deal of flexibility for states but then you have all these strings as to work participation requirements and who you can count which is turning

out to drive state behavior to a predictable but strong degree. (C. Miewald, personal interview, 1998)

Thus, we come to the central tension within the federal welfare legislation–states and localities have flexibility, but this flexibility is always constrained by both federal law and a public opinion that seems to promote a "work-first" approach. Contradictions emerge when the assumptions of the K-TAP program fail to meet with local economic and social conditions. Perhaps most problematic is the notion that poverty is due to individual decisions or choice. But as Garkovich et al. (1997, p. 2) note, in these places "there is an interaction among individuals and community characteristics that affect one's chances of being poor." A depressed economy, high rates of unemployment and poverty, a need for improved social services and a severe shortage of opportunities to earn a living wage are some of the conditions that make the emphasis on "work first" particularly difficult for Appalachian Kentuckians.

While much of the current welfare mythology is couched in terms of an urban underclass of welfare-dependent African-American and Latino families (Churchill, 1995), Appalachia has also been portrayed as a place of deviance from mainstream America (e.g., Shapiro, 1978). Appalachia has long served as the poster child for rural, white poverty and ascribed with many of the same "culture of poverty" characteristics assumed to exist in urban areas. Narratives that attempt to explain persistent poverty in the region often rely on viewing inhabitants as the dependent, uneducated and often pathological "Li'l Abner with a severely neurotic personality" (Banks et al., 1993, p. 295). But, as scholars of Appalachian history point out, it is the resource exploitation and large transfers of wealth out of the region, rather than the "culture of poverty," that is the cause of much of the region's economic problems (Billings and Tickamyer, 1993; Gaventa et al., 1996).

The people who live in the coal fields of Appalachian Kentucky have experienced decades of resource extraction, economic and political marginalization and persistent poverty and yet, they continue to survive. Welfare reform is only the latest in a long history of policies which have been imposed by outsiders who understood little about the culture, economics or politics of the region. At the same time, there is little doubt that welfare reform presents a new set of challenges for communities and there are those in the region that fear that the loss of federal assistance will result in the destruction of their way of life.

While the national discourse about public assistance continues to focus on individual behaviors or pathological "cultures of poverty," explanations that focus on structural issues and linkages may lead to critiques of the current system. In Appalachia, many residents realize that the consequences of welfare reform are a community-wide issue. The loss of revenue from reductions in transfer funds threatens the health of both families and the community. When women's work is taken out of the community and forced into the wage labor market, there are fewer people to care for children or the elderly. This loss to the local economy of care is feared to be substantial as both the young and old rely on women's labor for their health and well-being (see Miewald, 2000).

Further complicating this picture is the lack of living-wage jobs in the region. In Appalachian Kentucky communities, single mothers are expected to go to work in an economy where the real unemployment approaches 45 percent (Collins et al., 1996). Even with a job, people in the county have difficulty being "self-sufficient." Coal mining, once the dominant employer in the region, is being replaced by low-paying government and service sector employment. Few jobs pay more than minimum wage and it is rarer yet to find one that pays $13.00 an hour, which is what a single mother with two children must earn in rural Kentucky to be "self-sufficient" (Pearce, 2001).[1] Women, in particular, are frequently underemployed and therefore must rely on other forms of assistance to make ends meet (Collins et al., 1996). Finally, as a source of income, transfer payments comprise over a third of the income in the county, with K-TAP alone contributing over 2 million dollars annually (Kentucky Cabinet for Families and Children, 1997). County officials are concerned that if people lose their benefits or move from the region, there will be a resultant loss of income in an already-struggling economy.

Yet, welfare and poverty are economic issues, not simply ones of discourse, symbolism or myth. In order to create policy that addresses the needs of localities, both the public and policymakers require an alternative to the "culture of poverty" construct. Without the power to develop alternative representations of welfare, it is difficult for local groups to influence the process by which policy is formulated. Instead, they must wait for strategic openings within the decision-making process, although this usually occurs after policy has already been formulated (Churchill, 1995). Thus, it is important to examine the structural spaces or "cracks" within K-TAP where local power may be useful in challenging both welfare myths and policy. These spaces may emerge as opposition to attempts to move from a welfare to a workfare state, providing the possibility for new interpretations of the causes of poverty (Maxwell, 1996). The question for us today is whether the new institutional context of a reconfigured welfare system "yields the resources to participate in the creation of their own lives ... can it yield them power" (Piven 1996, p. 189).

Despite the apparent hegemony of welfare myths and the political marginalization of K-TAP participants, devolution and reconfiguration of public assistance has created unlikely allies and possibilities at the local level. County officials fearful of losing transfer payments, community colleges, which stand to see a decline in enrollment, and social service workers, whose jobs are threatened by privatization, find common ground with parents and welfare advocates in contesting state policy. As Piven (1990, p. 260) notes, the welfare system has "helped to create new solidarities and has also generated the political issues that cement and galvanize these solidarities." So too has the new emphasis on devolution. Piven (1996, p. 190) notes, "Even institutional arrangements that achieve social control are never entirely secure, for people discover new resources and evolve new ideas." The inclusion of "the local perspective" into the planning process has created new pathways for the inclusion of previously marginalized perspectives.

In Kentucky, however, there is a perception that the needs of the Appalachian region are given little weight in Frankfort. Appalachian residents often speak of two Kentuckys–the western half where all the political power and economic prosperity lay and the eastern side, which was either exploited or ignored. This sense of alienation is even more prevalent among K-TAP participants, most of whom are women with little experience in politics. For example, one K-TAP participant expressed her frustration that welfare reform did not appear to take the needs of people on welfare into account.

> People in Frankfort say they listen but I don't think they do because I think that unless you're in someone's situation, you don't understand where they're coming from. I think that a bunch of people in an office somewhere decided that we need welfare reform and we do, but they didn't talk to the people on welfare. They didn't ask us, what can we do to get you off? (C. Miewald, personal interview, 1997)

APPALSHOP:
LISTENING TO THE LIVED EXPERIENCE OF WELFARE

Since the effects of welfare policy are so wide, it is important to study it as a total social phenomenon that produces economic, legal, cultural, and moral implications that in turn can create new sets of relationships between communities, institutions and people (Shore and Wright, 1997, p. 7). The economic and social stress that welfare reform threatens to place on local institutions in Appalachian Kentucky has served to demystify policy and highlight the linkages between public assistance programs and community survival. Community members have come together to create the discursive 'space' to articulate their vision of welfare policy. It is in these "free spaces" that local concerns and experiences are expressed and "where participants can begin to see the connection between their concerns and those of other exploited people; where members can come to confront issues of racism and sexism; and where people can start to envision new alternatives to the world in which they live" (Fisher, 1993, p. 329, see also Couto, 1993 and Evans and Boyte, 1986).

Free space for participants to reshape welfare can be difficult to create, particularly in situations where overt class and gender inequalities limit access to the policy making process. Appalshop, a media collective based in Appalachian Kentucky, has produced one type of free space for the expression of local perspectives. Through community forums, film, and radio broadcasts, Appalshop has been applying "community-directed media" (Ruby 1992, p. 52) to issues of welfare policy. Mainstream media often limits public discourse because of its tendency to be produced "from the center," containing information that is non-local and decontextualized. Media which is both created by and reflective of a local community, however, produces spaces "at the margins" for new forms of knowledge and therefore is "subversive to the [homogenizing] intentions of most forms of mass media" (Ruby 1993, p. ix). Part of Appalshop's strategy for community development is to create public spaces where information and ideas can be exchanged. This flow of information enhances the possibility that Appalachian people can tell their own stories and solve their own problems, rather than relying on outside "experts" (Kirby, 1993).

In one town meeting, held at Appalshop, community members spoke to Minnesota Senator Paul Wellstone about their concerns with the effects of federal welfare policy on the region. The arrival of Senator Wellstone in Appalachian Kentucky provided an opportunity for residents to discuss their concerns with a member of Congress. While there were a number of issues raised in the course of the public forum, including mining conditions, water quality, and economic development, welfare reform was a central area of discussion. In particular, one longtime health and welfare rights activist stressed the importance of local experience in the production of state and national policy. She commented,

> Talking about welfare, I know all about it. Day after day I see the suffering of our people and I just wish the senators who pass these laws and make these bills could see it or have input from us, people that know what it's like to live on welfare . . . I just wish they would take the opportunity to come and listen to the cold, hard facts of life in Appalachia. (Appalshop, 1997)

In the forum and the subsequent radio spots, personal testimony challenged the "facts" of welfare as presented by politicians and the mainstream media–the problem is not a lack of a work ethic but the lack of jobs in the area. The solution is not more punitive policies that will cause additional hardship, but more opportunities for people to find living-wage jobs. For activists, it is this type of firsthand knowledge of welfare that can create serious holes in stereotypes and form the basis for more humane public policy. The question remains, however, whether local discursive spaces and value systems can be utilized in efforts to reformulate policy at the state and federal levels.

THE KENTUCKY WELFARE RIGHTS COALITION: TRANSLATING EXPERIENCE INTO POLICY

One effort to translate local needs to state government was undertaken last year by Kentucky Youth Advocates, a research and policy center concerned with the well-being of children, and Kentuckians for the Commonwealth (KFTC), an economic and social justice organization. In a series of community meetings, K-TAP participants and others were invited to share their stories about how welfare changes will affect them, their families and their communities. Appalshop filmed these meetings and segments were compiled into a short videotape that was disseminated to state legislators in order to undermine the "any job is a good job" rhetoric and provide support for pro-education legislation. One such story highlighted the frustration many K-TAP participants feel with the state's emphasis on work over education. As a 22-year-old mother and community college student stated,

> The choice I was given was either being abused or getting on welfare. I was a victim of domestic violence and my son a victim of child abuse and for me the only way out was to get on welfare. It's not fun going to the grocery store and paying for food with food stamps. It's one of the most embarrassing things that you can do.

[But] I would rather be on welfare and further my education so I could have a better job. (Quoted in Pickering, 1997)

This type of "back-talk" (see Stewart, 1990) challenges the political rhetoric that devalues the work of "getting an education," of "looking after the children" and of "keeping up the house" and reasserts these activities as necessary for the economic and social well-being of the community. It also provides a counter to all the negative images of welfare. As one K-TAP participant noted, the mainstream media only presents one picture of welfare.

You don't hear about the good things that people that draw welfare do, all you hear about is the bad stuff, the drug addicts and the people that steal food stamps and the old myth of the welfare Cadillac. You just don't hear about the others. (C. Miewald, personal interview, 1997)

However, simply challenging media stereotypes was often not enough for many K-TAP participants; they wanted to be directly involved in the creation of policy. After several months of discussion and negotiation, the Kentucky Welfare Reform Coalition, a diverse group of professional advocates, activists, and parents, agreed to create legislation that would provide additional educational opportunities for low-income people. One member of KWRC stressed the importance of moving beyond simply having parents tell their experiences and using those experiences in the creation of policy. In the effort to create public assistance legislation,

[K-TAP Parents] got organized and then they did some serious work on policies including some very detailed things that they wanted to see in the bill. One of the interesting things in all these discussions we had here was that as the policy wonk, I wasn't the one that was thinking in the greatest level of picky policy detail. Because parents had particular experiences and frustrations with programs they wanted to make sure some very detailed things got addressed in how those programs were run. (C. Miewald, personal interview, 1998)

Increased access to post-secondary education, the elimination of the 20-hour work requirement, the need for childcare and transportation and the development of advisory councils on each campus were among the policy changes proposed in the bill. While these policy changes reflected the needs of at least some K-TAP participants, the state balked at the creation of a separate state program using maintenance of effort money because of the fear that it may result in penalties from the federal level. In the end, a compromise was reached that would provide parents with support services and create an advisory council but will not stop the 5-year time clock or reduce the work requirement. House Bill 434, which was signed into law on April 1, 1998, reflects collaboration between policy-making and organizing efforts. Perhaps equally important was the demystification of the process by which policy is constructed for parent-activists. They were no longer solely the subjects of policymaking, but active participants in the process.

Given this example, we can perhaps be hopeful that there exist avenues within which local experience can make a difference in public policy. But for local experience to make a difference, it must be communicated, in a variety of ways, to other levels. Whether through media or working with state and national organizations, there is the need for the creation of linkages and alliances from the grassroots upward. Devolution has provided the opportunity for increased local-level decision-making and it is this privileging of "the local" that may provide a means to reconfigure welfare in ways that reflect knowledge and thoughtfulness rather than myth and rhetoric.

CONCLUSION

Welfare has different meanings for people who occupy differing social and economic positions. Within the current welfare debate, the voices of low-income parents have been marginalized because they lack political power. Furthermore, stigma associated with welfare means that low-income parents are often reluctant to participate in public discussions of or efforts to challenge existing policies. The result has been policy based upon what appear to be "rational" economic assessments and normative American cultural values, but which excludes the lived experience of low-income parents. The challenge for those advocating change is to find ways to transmit excluded discourses to politicians and the general public and to explore paths through which information can be used to subvert welfare myths. In the case I discuss in this paper, low-income women were able to tell their own stories about welfare using public spaces and media. In doing so, they articulated needs that are disallowed in the national rhetoric and state policy on public assistance. Stories that focus on the need for education, the value of providing care and the daily struggles of parents formed the basis for the creation of alternative public assistance policy.

For example, the use of media which is sensitive to community concerns can assist in the creation of information flows between federal, state and local scales, thereby contributing to the deconstruction of the welfare myth and the expansion of the realities upon which welfare policy is based. It can also create flows into the community, for the goal of improving awareness of state and federal policy. In other words, I suggest that the use of media can play a role in breaking down the barriers of socially produced geographical scales like "the local" and "the national" in order to facilitate a better understanding of the everyday experience of welfare. Such an understanding would enhance relationships between people's experience at the local scale and macro-level political-economic conditions that contextualize that experience. As anthropologists studying the reconfigurations of welfare, we must take seriously the potential for representational strategies to influence public policy and to recognize the varied ways in which local knowledge might be brought into the wider public sphere. We can assist this endeavor through the creation of ethnographic documentation of differential needs of the poor, objective effects of welfare policy and the role of human agency in reinterpreting both needs and policy (see Maxwell, 1996; Francis-Okongwu; 1996; Jarrett 1994).

Equally important are ways in which those directly affected by welfare's reconfiguration created their own spaces in which to challenge the assumptions upon which policy is based. The direct involvement of parents in the creation of HB 434 provides the important lesson that experience can be effectively translated into policy. Parents rejected the rhetoric and mythology of welfare and actively asserted their vision of a system, a vision that takes into account a diversity of situations and goals. Through their testimony and direct action, they offered a much-needed critique of the individualized and depoliticized framework that constitutes both myth and policy. In 1998, however, the question remained open as to whether local voices can make an ongoing difference in constructing public assistance policy. When asked if parents had the power to create a welfare system to meet their needs, one advocate responded, "Generally, I think we have a democracy, but it's an awful lot of work."

By 2002, a number of events support the argument that politicians and policymakers are listening to local concerns about welfare policy. In 1999, the Kentucky Cabinet for Families and Children announced that the state would allow 24 months of post-secondary education without any additional work requirement for full-time students. Furthermore, student-parents are able to count 10 hours per week of class time toward their 30-hour weekly work requirement.[2] In addition, the Cabinet now offers a $250 bonus to any participant who completes his or her education. The Cabinet, in conjunction with the Kentucky Community and Technical College System, has also developed the "Ready for Work" program through which case managers provide supportive services and facilitate work-study placements for the K-TAP students (for more on these programs, see Kentucky Cabinet for Families and Children 2001; Miewald, forthcoming). Those groups who worked on HB 434 have responded to these changes favorably. According to one assessment of K-TAP policies, Kentucky "used flexibility under the Temporary Assistance to Needy Families block grant to craft a mix of work, education and training activities for parents. In the process, the state became a recognized leader in affording access to post-secondary education" (Kentucky Youth Advocates, 2002, p. 1).

Yet, policies that address the needs of low-income parents are once again being threatened. As the reauthorization of welfare reform is being debated, there is the fear that proposed increases in participation rates will further erode the positive steps some states have made toward allowing access to education. According to a recent study, Kentucky would be one of the 40 states that would have to reduce access to education if participation rates were to increase (Center for Law and Social Policy, 2002). The challenge for welfare rights activists is to continue to find ways of breaking down the barriers to participation by those most directly affected by welfare's reconfigurations.

NOTES

1. The Self-Sufficiency Standard measures how much income is needed, for a family of a given composition in a given place, to adequately meet their basic needs without public or private assistance.

2. The change was possible only because Kentucky complied with federal welfare reform legislation that requires states to have an average of 25 percent of welfare recipients participating in a work activity.

REFERENCES

Albelda, R. and Tilly, C. (1996). It's a family affair: women, poverty and welfare. In A. Withorn (Ed.) *For crying out loud: women's poverty in the United States.* Boston: South End Press.

Appalshop (1997). Public forum with Senator Paul Wellstone. Transcript. Whitesburg, KY: Author.

Banks, A., Billings, D., and Tice, K. (1993). Appalachian studies, resistance, and postmodernism. In S.L Fisher (Ed) *Fighting back in Appalachia: traditions of resistance and change*. Philadelphia: Temple University Press.

Billings, D. and Tickamyer, A. (1993). Uneven development in Appalachia. In T.A. Lysona and W.W. Falk (Eds.), *Uneven development in rural America*. Lawrence: University Press of Kansas.

Center for Law and Social Policy (2002). Forty states likely to cut access to postsecondary training or education under House-passed bill. Available on-line *http://www.clasp.org/pubs/jobseducation/Postsec_survey_061902.htm*

Churchill, N. (1995). Ending welfare as we know it: a case study in urban Anthropology and public policy. *Urban Anthropology* 24(1-2), 5-35.

Collins, T., Eller, R., and Taul, G. (1996). *KRADD: historic trends and geographic patterns*. Lexington, KY: University of Kentucky Appalachian Center.

Couto, R. A. (1993). The memory of miners and the conscience of capital: coal miners' strikes as Free Spaces. In S.L Fisher (Ed.) *Fighting back in Appalachia: theories of resistance and change*. Philadelphia: Temple University Press.

Cerullo, M. and Erlien, M. (1996). Beyond the 'normal family': a cultural critique of women's poverty. In A. Withorn (Ed.) *For crying out loud: women's poverty in the United States*. Boston: South End Press.

Evans, S. M. and Boyte H.C. (1986). *Free spaces: the sources of democratic change in America*. New York: Harper and Row.

Flanders, L. (1996). Media lies: media, public opinion and welfare. In A. Withorn (Ed.) *For crying out loud: women's poverty in the United States*. Boston: South End Press.

Francis-Okongwu, A. (1995). Looking up from the bottom to the ceiling of the basement floor: female single-parent families surviving on $22,000 or less a year. *Urban Anthropology* 24, 313-362.

_____ (1996). Keeping the show on the road: female-headed families surviving on $22,000 a year or less in New York City. *Urban Anthropology* 25(2), 115-163.

Fraser, N. and Gordon, L. (1996). The genealogy of dependency: tracing a keyword in the U.S. welfare state. In A. Withorn (Ed.) *For crying out loud: women's poverty in the United States*. Boston: South End Press.

Garkovich, L., Hansen, G., and Dyk, P. (1997). Welfare reform and its implications for Kentucky's families on the economic edge. Lexington, KY: Cooperative Extension Service.

Gaventa, J., Smith B. E., and Willingham, A. (Eds.) (1990). Introduction. In *Communities in economic crisis: Appalachia and the South*. Philadelphia: Temple University Press.

Gilbert, M. (1997). Identity, space and politics: a critique of the poverty debates. In J.P. Jones, H. Nast and S. Roberts (Eds.) *Thresholds in feminist geography: difference, methodology and representation*. Lanham: Rowman and Littlefield.

Harvey, M., Summers, G., Pickering K., and Richards, P. (2002). The short-term impacts of welfare reform in persistently poor rural areas, In B. Weber, G. J. Duncan and L. A. Whitener (Eds.) *Rural dimensions of welfare reform*. Kalamazoo, MI: W.E. Upjohn Institute for Employment Research.

Jarrett, R. (1994). Living poor: family life among single-parent, African-American women. *Social Problems* 41(1), 30-49.

Kentucky Cabinet for Families and Children (1996). *Kentucky Transitional Assistance Program (K-TAP)*. Frankfort, KY: Cabinet for Families and Children.
_____ (1997). *Statewide data book*. Frankfort, KY.
_____ (2001). *Temporary Assistance for Needy Families (TANF) State Plan–Kentucky*. Available on-line at *http://cfc.state.ky.us/reform/reform.asp*
Kentucky Youth Advocates (2001). *Kentucky welfare reform assessment project*. Available on-line at *http://www.kyyouth.org/Publications/kwrap1.pdf*
Kirby, R. (1993). Radio and the distribution of power in Central Appalachia. In H. Mowlana and M.H. Frondorf (Eds.), *The media as a forum for community building: cases from Africa, Latin America, Eastern Europe and the United States*. Baltimore: The Johns Hopkins University.
Kyl, J. (1995). Welfare reform: common sense solutions to the welfare crisis. Testimony before the Senate, Aug. 8. Washington, D.C.: THOMAS: U.S. Congress on the Internet.
Lexington Herald-Leader (1997). Many counties unprepared for welfare reform: clock ticking for recipients to find jobs. June 19. A1. Lexington, KY.
Maxwell, A. (1996). "Human rights and social welfare policy reform views from the field": a discussion. *Urban Anthropology* 25(2), 211-219.
Miewald, C.E. (2000). Women's work? Caring, kinship and community in Appalachian Kentucky. Unpublished Dissertation. Lexington, KY: University of Kentucky.
_____ (Forthcoming). "This little light of mine": parent-activists struggling for access to post-secondary education in Appalachian Kentucky, In P. Kahn, S. Butler, L. Deprez, V. Polakow (Eds.) *Parenting, work and education: low-income mothers in post-secondary education*. New York: SUNY Press.
Mink, G. (1998). *Welfare's end*. Ithaca: Cornell University Press.
Oliker, S. (1995a). The proximate contests of workfare and work: a framework for studying poor women's economic choices. *The Sociological Quarterly* 36(2), 251-272.
_____ (1995b). Work commitment and constraint among mothers on workfare. *Journal of Contemporary Ethnography* 24(2), 165-194.
Pearce, D. (with J. Brooks) (2001). *The self-sufficiency standard for Kentucky: real budgets, real families*. Louisville, KY: Kentucky Youth Advocates.
Peck, J. (1996). Permeable welfare? Workfare politics and the deconstruction of Canada's work-welfare regime. Paper presented at the conference Crisis of Global Regulation and Governance, Athens, GA, April 6-8, 1996.
_____ (1998). Postwelfare Massachusetts. *Economic Geography*, Special Issue for the 1998 Annual Meeting of the Association of American Geographers, 62-82.
Pickering, M. (1997). *Testimony on education and welfare reform*. Video recording. Whitesburg, KY: Appalshop.
Piven, F. (1996). Women and the state: ideology, power and welfare. In L. Gordon (Ed.) *Women, the state and welfare*. Madison: University of Wisconsin Press.
Piven, F. and Cloward, R. (1997). *The breaking of the American social compact*. New York: The New Press.
Schram, S. (2000). *After welfare: the culture of postindustrial social policy*. New York University Press.
Seccomb, K. (1999). *So you think I drive a Cadillac? Welfare recipients' perspectives on the system and its reform*. Boston: Allyn and Bacon.

Shore, C. and Wright, S. (1997). Policy: A new field of Anthropology. In C. Shore and S. Wright (Eds.) *Anthropology of policy: critical perspectives on governance and power*, London: Routledge.

Shapiro, H. D. (1978). *Appalachia on our mind: the Southern mountains and mountaineers in the American consciousness, 1870-1920*. Chapel Hill: University of North Carolina Press.

Shaw, C. Jr. (1996). Supporting true welfare reform. Testimony before the House of Representatives, extension of remarks, May 22. Washington, D.C. THOMAS: U.S. Congress on the Internet.

Stewart, K. (1990). Backtalking the wilderness: Appalachian en-genderings. In F. Ginsburg and A.T. Tsing (Eds.) *Uncertain terms: negotiating gender in American culture*, Boston: Beacon Press.

Thomas, S. L. (1997). Women, welfare, reform and the preservation of a myth. *The Social Science Journal* 34 (3), 351-368.

THOUGHTS ON POVERTY AND INEQUALITY

Driving Out of Poverty in Private Automobiles

Lisa M. Brabo
Peter H. Kilde
Patrick Pesek-Herriges
Thomas Quinn
Inger Sanderud-Nordquist

SUMMARY. Transportation is a critical problem for Welfare-to-Work households; thus, the West Central Wisconsin Community Action

Agency, Inc. developed resources to launch a facilitated-automobile purchase program named JumpStart. The program data and client survey results presented in this paper show that ownership of a private automobile is a key element of success in Welfare-to-Work households in rural areas. Private automobiles make it possible for families to obtain the "assets" of independence: job training or education, a good job, health care, child care, social supports, and even self-esteem and family/community relationships. *[Article copies available for a fee from The Haworth Document Delivery Service: 1-800-HAWORTH. E-mail address: <docdelivery@haworthpress.com> Website: <http://www.HaworthPress.com> © 2003 by The Haworth Press, Inc. All rights reserved.]*

KEYWORDS. Welfare, transportation, poverty, rural

INTRODUCTION AND OVERVIEW

West CAP (the West Central Wisconsin Community Action Agency, Inc.) is a community-based organization operating in a 7-county area proximate to the twin cities of Minneapolis and St. Paul, Minnesota. In 1998, administrators of the organization developed hypotheses regarding the transportation problems of Welfare-to-Work households in a rural area. It was believed that only the private automobile could meet all of the needs of TANF or Wisconsin Works (W-2) households.

The agency developed resources to launch a facilitated-automobile purchase program named JumpStart. The program provides down payment loans and case management support. At the date of this paper, JumpStart has helped 90 eligible households purchase late-model, warranted automobiles. In order to provide low-interest loans to clients, West CAP developed partnerships with credit unions, obtaining preferential interest rates. In order to provide the lowest possible prices, the agency took the innovative step of becoming an automobile dealer, able to purchase at wholesale automobile auctions.

Evaluation of the program shows that combined interest and price savings average $3,900 per client household, and that the program provides its services at reasonable public cost. A survey of clients owning program vehicles for 6 months or more provides evidence of success in terms of the job income development purposes of the program. In fact, the program data and client survey results presented in this paper argue strongly that ownership of a private automobile is a key element of success in obtaining the "assets" of independence: job training or education, a good job, health care, child care, social supports, and even self-esteem and family/community relationships.

THE PROBLEM

When America set out to replace welfare with work, it was generally recognized that the transportation needs of new workers would have to be met in order for this reform policy to succeed. Four years after the full implementation of welfare reform, the lack of an adequate transportation solution has emerged as one of the most intractable barriers to the integration of former AFDC recipients into the work force.

As we better understand the direct experiences of TANF recipients in moving into the workforce, the full dimensions of this transportation barrier are more fully appreciated. Recent studies in Minnesota provide a good example. A May 2001 report by the Hennepin County Planning Department looked at several recent studies on transportation needs in the Minneapolis/St. Paul metropolitan area (*Transportation and Low Income Workers*, 2001). These studies clearly identified transportation as the greatest obstacle for welfare recipients in finding or keeping a job. The primary finding was that while half of the people on welfare live in the core city, seventy percent of the jobs available to them are located in the suburbs. Three-quarters of the welfare recipients reported that they must rely on public transit to get to their jobs. The studies showed that few of these jobs are sufficiently clustered to support the provision of frequent public transit service, or to address the irregular transportation needs frequently encountered by persons working entry-level jobs (evening, night or weekend shifts).

The report also reviewed a study by three county-sponsored group transportation partnerships. In the partnerships' own words:

> All of the group transportation pilot programs, including van pooling and mini-route buses, were unsuccessful. Despite extensive efforts to recruit employers and riders from a sizable (TANF) population, limited ridership made group transportation strategies cost-ineffective.

The Hennepin County report cited partnership strategies that did demonstrate success, all of which were focused on private vehicle access and maintenance. For example, a program that offered gap services consisting of car donations combined with supportive assistance for repair, insurance and maintenance costs had the highest rate for movement of participants out of welfare and into unsubsidized work. In 2000, approximately 68% of participants who received this kind of vehicle assistance were able to obtain or retain employment, and 14% moved out of welfare.

Although this report of studies addresses an urban situation, where it is at least possible to consider fundamental changes in transportation policies that could provide long-term solutions (e.g., public investment in transit; transportation management strategies) the results are nevertheless informative for welfare-to-work programs in rural areas. If it is difficult to make public and group transit programs work efficiently in densely populated urban areas, it is not surprising that the same project is nearly impossible in rural areas, where the population is dispersed and public transit is practically nonexistent. Alternately, if ownership of private vehicles is a workable remedy in urban areas, this approach is even more likely to be workable in rural areas. Over 65% of rural Americans live in areas with either no public transit service or very negligible transit service (*Benefits of Rural Transportation*, 1998). Even in areas with service, it is likely to focus on fairly specific or high priority needs: the elderly, disabled, special medical concerns.

In most cases, service quality is difficult and expensive to maintain. Most of these services are provided by vans (53%) or small buses (21%) that have restricted operating times and destinations. Half of these vehicles are considered to be past their life expectancies; 60% are not wheelchair accessible. Limited resources are also a problem.

The unfortunate result is that, as one study observed, while "almost 1,200 public transportation systems exist in rural communities across the U.S.; no single transportation strategy appropriately addresses the diversity of rural America" (*Benefits of Rural Transportation*, 1998).

For low-income persons, ownership of personal vehicles is every bit as great a problem. In 1995 only 4% of non-low-income U.S. households did not own a car, compared with 24% of low-income households. From another perspective, approximately 62% of all U.S. households who do not own autos can be considered poor or "near poor" (*Nationwide Personal Transportation Survey*, 1990 and 1995). The numbers for rural areas, taken discretely, are similar. While about 7% of rural households do not have cars, the proportion rises to 57% for rural poor–an especially troubling number given the limited availability of rural transit (*Benefits of Rural Transportation*, 1998).

In 1999 and 2000, the Wilder Research Foundation conducted an assessment of the quality of life in the St. Croix River Valley (the counties of Washington in Minnesota and Pierce, Polk and St. Croix in Wisconsin). These counties comprise suburban, ex-urban and rural areas that share the commonality of the St. Croix River watershed. The study, funded by the Hugh J. Andersen Foundation, included a first phase that compiled available demographic, social and economic information and, in the fall of 2000, a survey of 1,612 residents, conducted by telephone. The first phase data compilation clearly established the absence of public transit, particularly in the rural Wisconsin counties, and the high incidence of commuting. In the three Wisconsin counties, there were 3 "public transit facilities" (1 in Pierce, 2 in St. Croix)–all of which were municipally-based taxi services. All the Wisconsin counties had more commuters traveling to Minnesota (16,527 people) than coming from Minnesota (3,686 people), and two of the counties (Pierce and Polk) had more net commuter travel to other Wisconsin counties (*Lay of the Land*, 1999).

The Y2000 Wilder survey again established high rates of commuting. A net of 42.6% of respondents (N = 1168) said that they commute 30 or more miles round trip for work (*St. Croix Valley*, 2001). (Travel to work of less than 15 miles each way was not counted as commuting.) How do they commute, in a situation where public transit is virtually nonexistent? The survey reported that 97% of residents rely on their own cars for all transportation.

The West CAP Transportation Program

It may be self-evident that work-related transportation is a special challenge for low-income households with children as they leave dependency on welfare and seek to enter the work force–especially in a rural area. The West Central Wisconsin Community Action Agency, Inc. attempted to inventory the transportation needs of these households and to develop a demonstration program to meet those needs. The first step was to establish the criteria for an acceptable transportation program, thereby developing a hypothesis for a workable program. The second step was to implement that program and test its results.

Criteria and Hypothesis: Becky Gets to Work

During the 60-year life span of AFDC, American life has developed around the assumption that everybody has a car. Over time, the ideal model of neighborhoods and communities where work, groceries, dry goods, school, church, medical care, medicine, family and friends are all within walking distance of home has virtually disappeared. In light of this reality, West CAP posited the minimum transportation needs of a typical single working mother in today's economy. They named her "Becky," and constructed her story.

> Becky received AFDC for a while, before it was eliminated by the 1997 federal TANF legislation. Now she works, earning just enough to keep her family together–so long as she receives subsidized childcare and Medicaid (no health insurance at her job). Her days are filled with travel: early in the morning, she takes 3-year-old Sam to the Warm World Day Care Center and 6-year-old Danielle to school. Then she drives to work. During lunch, she often runs the kinds of errands every mother knows: getting a prescription filled, finding the right notebook for Danielle, getting her uniform from the dry cleaner. After work, she picks up the kids, goes home to cook, plays with the children until bedtime, and maybe kicks back with a late-night TV program. On weekends, she does the grocery shopping, looks for bargains at the Goodwill store, goes to the laundromat, has an outing with her sister's family, or brings the kids to the park. A couple times a year she likes to get back to her folks in Iowa and connect Sam and Danielle to that part of their family history.

In a very real sense, Becky's situation is representative of the unprecedented transportation challenge facing post-welfare America at the beginning of a new century. There is no real-life bus that fits Becky's needs. There will be no such bus in the reasonable future. To be successful–to support basic family activities and provide an opportunity to advance in the workforce–any transportation solution must at least meet the modest needs of families such as Becky's. At the same time, any enduring transportation solution for these families must be accountable to public policy concerns about cost-effectiveness and environmental sustainability. In its literature, West CAP argued that conventional programs fail both the needs test and the test of cost-effectiveness.

West CAP's Criteria

Every family situation is unique, but we believe that a transportation solution that meets Becky's needs would likely work in most situations–rural and urban. What are the *minimum* transportation requirements of this family?

1. *Safety.* Beyond getting herself to work, Becky transports the most precious cargo in the world, and transports them a lot. In addition to round trips to day care and school, the kids are along on errands, appointments and recreational outings.
2. *Reliability.* Becky needs to get to work, day care, and school 5 days out of every week, in rain, shine, snow, sub-zero temperatures, or whatever. There are doctor's appointments, minor emergencies, and a very hectic every day schedule.
3. *Flexibility.* The complexity of Becky's schedule on even a "normal" day requires great flexibility, both in terms of the places Becky and the kids have to go and when they have to be there–and, of course, in the real world every day is not normal.
4. *Manageability.* Take the transportation demands under Flexibility and try to imagine meeting them while depending on volunteer drivers. Now try city buses, car pools, van pools, taxis, trains, or bicycles. Now try it in a rural area.
5. *Affordability.* Becky's budget is tight and will remain tight for a long time. When and if her income rises, so will her childcare co-payments. No real progress will be made in her standard of living until she is earning over $12.00/hr.
6. *Consistent, Predictable Monthly Expenses.* Becky's tight budget means that her transportation cannot surprise her with a large unexpected cost such as a transmission failure, the unplanned necessity to replace a car, or even a more modest repair.
7. *Long-Term Function.* Becky's climb up the ladder and out of poverty will be a long climb. A short-term transportation solution may not suffice. If she falls off the ladder because of transportation problems, she may be in a worse situation than she was on AFDC, with less time on her clock and another failure on her mind.
8. *Rural and Urban Applicability.* Many former AFDC recipients live in rural communities with limited or nonexistent public transportation. Even inner-city workers are finding that relying on public transit can limit their access to better paying jobs.
9. *Reasonable Public Cost.* Continued public support will be essential to the success of any transportation program that meets the needs of families like Becky's, but these public costs will need to be perceived as reasonable, efficient, and affordable.
10. *Environmental Sustainability.* An enduring transportation solution for low-income families must also address issues of environmental sustainability, and should demonstrate the use of energy saving strategies and new technologies. Low-income families should play a leading role in the development of these options.

West CAP's analysis led to the conclusion that the private automobile is the only workable transportation program for its rural community. West CAP set itself the task of funding and demonstrating a program of facilitated automobile purchase for TANF-eligible households. To do this, West CAP established partnerships with six county TANF management agencies (W-2 agencies, in Wisconsin's vernacular) and with an area credit union. Funding from the state of Wisconsin, from the county W-2 agencies, and from the Otto Bremer Foundation initiated and sustained the program. Since March 1999, when the first car purchase was made, West CAP has operated the JumpStart program of facilitated automobile purchase which, the organization believes, has demonstrated the ability to meet all of the transportation needs of its clientele.

THE JUMPSTART PROGRAM

West CAP's JumpStart program helps its clients purchase late-model, warranted automobiles that meet minimum thresholds for efficiency and safety. The agency believes that its program's emphasis on fuel efficiency also provides a model for movement toward environmental sustainability.

The JumpStart program has three interrelated components: (1) client relationships, including outreach, assessment, and support, (2) financing partnerships with local lending institutions, and (3) an "in-house" automobile dealership license, with an experienced automobile buyer.

JumpStart participants are TANF eligible households (under 200% of poverty, with children) whose situations have been evaluated by W-2 Financial and Employment Planners (FEPs). Program staff members work with each family to evaluate their transportation needs and their credit worthiness.

In partnership with one of the two participating local credit unions, they are able to create viable car purchase arrangements for eligible participants. In view of the financial evaluations by county FEPs and the case management support of JumpStart program staff, the credit unions offer JumpStart clients preferential interest rates–the same rates they charge their most credit-worthy clients. The value of this credit differential is significant, and will be discussed later in this report.

In order to provide the best possible prices to their clients, and to assure vehicle quality, West CAP has taken the innovative step of becoming a licensed automobile dealer. The dealership enables the program to purchase quality cars meeting program standards for efficiency and reliability directly from wholesale auctions, resulting in significant discounts. A typical JumpStart vehicle would be a two- or three-year-old Saturn or Geo Prizm with less than 40,000 miles, still covered by the factory warranty.

West CAP provides $3,000 for the client to use as a down payment loan, and works with the credit union to provide a low interest loan for the balance. The average of credit union loans has been approximately $5,000; clients make their payments on loans directly to the credit union. The $3,000 West CAP down payment portion is managed as a no interest "patient loan"; clients pay $25 each month directly to West CAP. If they successfully complete payment of their car loan during a 5-year amortization period, West CAP will forgive the remaining $1,500 of its down payment loan.

At the time of the purchase, and as a requirement of the down payment loan, West CAP establishes a contract between client and program, requiring the client to maintain insurance, agree to own no other vehicles, maintain a good driving record, make timely car payments, and provide for regular vehicle maintenance. Additionally, each car loan includes the purchase of a six-year/100,000 mile extended warranty that provides protection against the possibility of major repair costs. The dealership license allows purchase of this warranty at a discounted price (currently, $790). The JumpStart case manager is available to help with decision-making on these and related matters, throughout the client's participation in the program.

EVALUATION OF THE JUMPSTART PROGRAM

JumpStart Benefits: Program Data

At the date of this writing, the JumpStart program has helped 90 TANF/W-2 households purchase automobiles. Only two of the automobiles (2.2%) have had to be repossessed by the lending institution, and another two clients have voluntarily surrendered their cars owing to significant changes in their personal lives. The average retail value of the automobiles purchased is about $10,400. Low-income households have been able to afford these purchases for three significant reasons:

1. Down payment loans of $3,000 provided by the JumpStart program through its funding by state and local government and the Otto Bremer Foundation;

2. Price reductions that were initially gained through dealer discounts and are now obtained through the wholesale-purchasing abilities of the West CAP dealership;
3. Preferential interest rates provided by the collaborating area credit unions.

Down Payment Loans

As noted in the foregoing program description, the program provides a partially forgivable down payment loan of $3,000. At the repayment rate of $25 per month, clients who successfully complete the program, having paid off their credit union loan, will have repaid one-half the down payment loan. The balance of $1,500 will be forgiven.

Wholesale Prices

Against an average retail value of $10,400 (without extended warranty), the program has provided vehicles to its clients at an actual average cost of $8,000, which includes the cost of the extended warranty ($790). The average price-reduction saving per client has been $2,400. This purchase strategy also allows control over car quality and fuel efficiency. The fuel economy rating of cars purchased through JumpStart is over 32 mpg.

Preferred Interest Rates

High-risk borrowers are normally charged an 18% interest rate. Through the agreements negotiated by West CAP staff, JumpStart borrowers are receiving the same rate as the most credit-worthy borrowers served by the credit unions: 7.5% to 8%. This means that on a typical vehicle with an extended warranty financed at $5,000 (the balance remaining after West CAP's down payment loan), a JumpStart borrower is able to save over $1,500 on interest payments to the credit union during the five-year loan amortization period.

JumpStart staff collaborate with lenders on a policy requiring a household budget for each client. This client support, along with the regular monitoring procedures by the staff, means that JumpStart loans have a high probability of success. In fact, despite the poor initial credit rating of typical JumpStart clients, WESTconsin Credit Union reports that the delinquency rate on JumpStart loans is lower than the overall rate for their regular borrowers. This experience is having an impact on the credit policies of the lenders.

Public Costs

JumpStart is proving to be a fiscally prudent use of government funding. Of the $3,000 provided for the down payment loan, $1,500 is paid back by the client and is available to help additional clients. Of the remaining $1,500 in program assistance, $500 is returned to the state as sales tax on date of the purchase. The balance of $1000 is the net *direct* financial support to the participant household over the five-year period of the program loan.

There are, of course, *indirect* benefits to clients, in the form of supportive case management and program administration. Case management services include household financial management, liaison to other supportive services, support for job development, and consultation on vehicle maintenance. Administrative costs include supervision, accounting and audit. The current year's budget and vehicle purchase goals can be used as a base for calculating indirect support. The total JumpStart budget is $388,600. Of this amount, $148,000 is budgeted for down payment loans and a loan reserve fund. The balance of $240,600 serves the 50 clients of the current year, plus the 40 clients from the prior year (90 total). Thus, the cost-per-client for indirect support is just about $2,600. As client numbers increase–along with the relative self-sufficiency of clients–this cost will decrease.

West CAP believes that these costs represent a good investment in support of clients' efforts to obtain, retain, or improve employment, escape dependency on public benefits, and achieve self-sufficiency.

CLIENT SURVEY

Method

In order to evaluate the experience of the program in the lives of its clients, West CAP conducted a survey of all clients who had owned a JumpStart vehicle for 6 months or more. The survey was conducted by telephone during November 2001. The JumpStart program Special Projects Analyst attempted to contact 43 clients who had owned their cars for at least six months. Thirty-four clients were interviewed–79% of the target population. Those contacted were asked 14 questions as to their social and economic status and their program experience. Each set of responses was recorded by the interviewer. Responses were then entered into an SPSS database for analysis.

Findings

Of the 34 responding clients who owned JumpStart program automobiles for six months or more:

- 85% are employed, with 6% of these being self-employed. Twelve percent (12%) cannot work because of their own medical condition or that of a close family member for whom they give constant care
- Of those employed, the average wage is $9.80 per hour, approximately $2.00 per hour more than the average reported for employed TANF recipients in the same service area as served by the JumpStart program (Wisconsin Department of Workforce Development, 2001)
- Their average roundtrip commute is 24 miles
- Of those able to work, 53% have changed jobs since getting their JumpStart car
  - Of those, 100% report getting a better job
  - 75% report higher wages
  - 88% report that the JumpStart car helped them get their better job
- 53% report that transportation had been their biggest barrier in getting a better job, while an additional 18% shared transportation barriers equally with a second variable, such as education or lack of stable housing
- 79% report that there is no public transportation available to them
  - Of the remaining 21%, 86% report that the public transportation in their area cannot meet their needs
- 74% receive some sort of public assistance
  - Of those, 36% report that the level of assistance they receive has decreased since they received their JumpStart car
  - 50% credit the car with the reduction in other public assistance
- Of the 55% who have changed day care providers since getting their car
  - 100% report improved quality of day care
  - 50% credit their JumpStart car with their ability to access higher quality day care services
- 47% have advanced their formal education or technical training since acquiring their automobiles.
- 35% have moved since getting their car
  - Of those, 58% went from renting to home ownership

- 85% report improved credit ratings
- 68% report overall improved financial health
- 74% report more involvement with extended family, friends and community
- 100% report a better overall quality of life; 79% say it is much better
- Asked to rate the JumpStart program on a scale of one to ten with one being lousy and ten being outstanding:
  - 62% gave JumpStart a "10"
  - 23% gave it a "9," and 15% gave it an "8"
- All vehicles are now fully insured, over/against 54% prior to the program, demonstrating a clear social benefit in lowering the insurance risk to the public.
- In the majority of cases, older unsafe and inefficient vehicles have been removed from service and replaced by safe, efficient vehicles. West CAP has not yet developed a quantitative measure of these safety and efficiency achievements, but they appear to be substantial.

CONCLUSION

The JumpStart program responds to the transportation needs of TANF households moving from welfare to work by helping them purchase late-model, economical, dependable automobiles. This strategy is designed to provide transportation that is safe, reliable, flexible, affordable, sustainable, and cost-effective for the client and in terms of public policy. The private automobile was determined to be the only program that could meet all the transportation criteria for "Becky," the typical TANF head-of-household.

The program data and client survey results presented in this paper argue strongly that the program has succeeded in its purpose and that, in fact, ownership of a private automobile is a key element of success in obtaining the "assets" of independence: job training or education, a good job, health care, child care, social supports, and even self-esteem and family/community relationships.

While much of JumpStart's success rests on the development of practical tools that meet real-life needs–financing partnerships, car purchasing assistance, targeted subsidies and efficient case management–it is important to recognize that its success is also based on offering meaningful and realizable incentives to participants. For most Americans, poor and not poor, owning a good-quality, dependable automobile is not only a practical necessity and the key to gaining remunerative work; it is also a key to acceptance and participation in the social fabric of their community life.

JumpStart works as an incentive program because it connects participants to both their work and "the rest of life"–family visits, medical and other service appointments, shopping, school activities, etc. The program's focus on car quality and long-term support distinguish it from most other car-based programs that primarily assist with low-end purchases, or even donations, and offer little assurance of dependability. JumpStart derails the fairly common opinion that welfare households cannot (and perhaps *should not*–an attitude sometimes encountered) sustain the ownership of a good quality late model car. From the first day they drive their car, and the first month they make a loan payment, JumpStart participants experience a meaningful improvement in the quality of their lives.

REFERENCES

Transportation and Low Income Workers. (2001). Taskforce on Homeless Families, Hennepin County.
Benefits of Rural Transportation. (1998). Washington, DC: National Association of Development Organizations.
Nationwide Personal Transportation Survey. (1990 and 1995). Washington, DC: Bureau of Transportation Statistics.
Lay of the Land: Community Needs and Resources. (1999). St. Paul, MN: Wilder Research Center.
St. Croix Valley: Survey of Residents. (2001). St. Paul, MN: Wilder Research Center.
Wisconsin Department of Workforce Development. (2001). Madison, WI: State of Wisconsin.

Index

ACEnet, 135
Addams, J., 53
Adult(s), nonaged, in U.S., economic well-being of. *See also* Nonaged adults in United States, economic well-being of, gender differences in gender differences in, 97-122
AFDC. *See* Aid to Families with Dependent Children (AFDC)
Age, as factor in economic well-being in U.S., gender differences in, 97-122. *See also* Nonaged adults in United States, economic well-being of, gender differences in
Aid to Families with Dependent Children (AFDC), 3,9,32,35,43,53-54,64, 100,101,142-143,145,188
Albelda, R., 166
AMA. *See* American Medical Association (AMA)
"American Dream," 129
American Health Security Act plan, 16
American Medical Association (AMA), 13-14
American workers, real average hourly earnings of, 27,28f
Andreson, T., 136
Appalachia, Central, 123-139. *See also* Central Appalachia
Appalachian Cooperative Exchange Network (ACEnet), 135
Appalachian Kentucky
 described, 164
 policy creation in, 163-181
 introduction to, 164-165

Appalachian poverty, 124
Appalachian Regional Commission, 5, 127
Appalshop, 172-174
Arrow, K., 29

Bartle, E., 5,141
Bassuk, S.S., 144,145
Battle of Blair Mountain, 129
Becker, G.S., 118
Billings, D., 124,132
Blank, R., 36
Blee, K., 124,132
Bluegrass music, 136
Boeing, 39
Brabo, 5
Brabo, L.M., 183
Bronfenbrenner, K., 39-40
Browne, A., 144,145
Browne, W.P., 131
Buffalo Creek, flooding of, 132
Bureau of Justice Statistics, 144
Bush, G.W., Pres., 4,31,34

California Work Opportunity and Responsibility to Kids Program (CalWORKS), 5,147-148
 study of
  fear and distrust of caseworkers and system in general in, 155-157
  findings of, 149-158

good caseworkers in, 154-155
help from advocates other
than CalWORKS
caseworkers in,
152-154
insufficient and insensitive
information from
CalWORKS
caseworkers in,
150-152
methodology in, 148-149
sample in, 149
suggestions to improve
information given
by caseworkers in,
157-158
CalWORKS. *See* California Work
Opportunity and
Responsibility to Kids
Program (CalWORKS)
CalWORKS/TANF, 141
Census Bureau, 2
Center for Urban Research and
Learning, Loyola University,
6
Center on Budget and Policy Priorities,
56
Central Appalachia, 123-139
"culture of poverty" in, 132-134
future of, 135-136
government mistrust in, 129-130
poor of, described, 125-126
poverty in
historical background of,
127-129
invisibleness of, 131-132
reasons for, 127
progress in, forms of, 134-135
ruralness of, 130-131
vs. Southern Appalachia, 130
WASPS of, 125
Child Protective Services, 160
Children, effect on economic
well-being of nonaged adults
in U.S., 100

Children's Health Insurance Program
(CHIP), 15,30
CHIP. *See* Children's Health Insurance
Program (CHIP)
Civil War, 127
Clinton, B., Pres., 28,36-37,38,52,54
fair record of, 30-32
Clinton boom, staying poor in, 23-49
introduction to, 24-28,25f, 28f
Clinton plan, 13,17,18
Cloward, R., 166-167
Colamosca, A., 42
College of Arts and Sciences, Georgia
State University, 6
College of Social Work, Ohio State
University, 6
Compensator(s), and targeted policies,
30-32
Congress on Racial Equality (CORE),
127
Congressional Research Service, 101
Corbin, D., 129
Corcoran, M.E., 99
CORE. *See* Congress on Racial
Equality (CORE)
Cornelius, L.J., 3,7,17
Courant, P.En., 99
CPSs. *See* Current Population Surveys
(CPSs)
Critical discourse analysis (CDA),
56-57
Critical theory, 56
"Culture of poverty," in Central
Appalachia, 132-134
Cunningham, R., 125
Current Population Surveys (CPSs),
101

DeLong, B., 38
Department of Health and Human
Services (DHHS), 145,146
DHHS. *See* Department of Health and
Human Services (DHHS)
Domestic violence, 144-146

"Don't Feed the Alligators," 32
Douglass, F., 53
Duncan, C.M., 130
Duncan, G., 99

Earned Income Tax Credit (EITC), 30-31
Economic well-being, of nonaged adults in U.S., gender differences in, 97-122. *See also* Nonaged adults in United States, economic well-being of, gender differences in
Eisenhower, D.D., Pres., 37
EITC. *See* Earned Income Tax Credit (EITC)
Elderly, poverty among, 2
Exxon, 39

Family and Medical Leave Act of 1993, 119
Family Violence Option (FVO), 144, 145, 146, 148
Farmer, S.M., 127
Federal Reserve Board (FRB), 27, 37-38, 39, 42-43
FEPs. *See* Financial and Employment Planners (FEPs)
Financial and Employment Planners (FEPs), 190
Fisher's Exact Test, 74
"Fixing that Great Hodgepodge," 3-4
Foucault, M., 52, 56
Fourth World Conference on Women, 98
Fraser, N., 168
FRB. *See* Federal Reserve Board (FRB)
Freire, P., 52

FVO. *See* Family Violence Option (FVO)

GAIN, 152, 153, 160
Gans, H.J., 98
Garkovich, L., 170
Gingrich, N., 32
Gordon, L., 168
Government, mistrust of, in Central Appalachia, 129-130
Great Depression, 4, 53, 126
Greenspan, A., 29, 36, 37

Haber, S., 100
Habermas, J., 52
Halperin, R.H., 132
Halvorsen, R., 107, 108
Harrington, M., 2, 5, 8, 24, 52, 53, 123, 124, 125, 132, 142
Harris poll, 41
Hatch, O., 30
HB 434, 177, 178
Health care, for poor in U.S., 7-21
Health care coverage, before War on Poverty, 8
Health Security Act, 13
Hennepin County Planning Department, 185
Hill, M., 100
Hill-Burton program, 8
Hoffman, S., 99
Holahan, J., 11
Hong, B.E., 99
Hot Tuna, 136
House Energy and Commerce Committee, 14
House of Representatives, 4, 52
H&R Block, 37

Inequality, poverty and, 28-30
in U.S., introduction to, 1-6

Institute for Women's Policy
    Research, 145

Johnson, L.B., Pres., 98
Jordan, M., 29
Journal of Poverty, 6
*Journal of Poverty: Innovations on
    Social, Political & Economic
    Inequalities,* 53
JumpStart program, 184,190-191
    benefits of, 191-192
    case manager in, 191
    client survey related to, 193-195
    described, 184,190-191
    down payment loans from, 192
    evaluation of, 191-193
    preferred interest rates in, 192-193
    public costs of, 193
    Special Projects Analysis of,
        193-194
    wholesale prices through, 192
JumpStart vehicle, typical, 191

Kamerman, S.B., 11
Kaukonen, J., 136
Kendall's tau, 74
Kennedy, T., 30
Kentuckians for the Commonwealth
    (KFTC), 174
Kentucky, Appalachian, policy
    creation in, 163-181
Kentucky Cabinet for Families and
    Children, 177
Kentucky Community and Technical
    College System, 178
Kentucky Transitional Assistance
    Program (K-TAP), 164
    described, 169-172
Kentucky Welfare Rights Coalition
    (KWRC), 174-176
Kerr-Mills program, 8

KFTC. *See* Kentuckians for the
    Commonwealth (KFTC)
Kilde, P.H., 183
Kilty, K.M., 1,2,4,51
K-TAP. *See* Kentucky Transitional
    Assistance Program (K-TAP)
KWRC. *See* Kentucky Welfare Rights
    Coalition (KWRC)
Kyl, J., Sen., 168

Labor force, hidden, 36-42
Labor markets, ignoring of, 32-36
Lamas, E., 100
Landes, M., 118
Lewis, O., 132
Live from Fur Peace Ranch, 136

Madrick, J., 29
Malthus, T., 53
Marital status, effect on economic
    well-being of nonaged adults
    in U.S., 99-100
Matewan Massacre, 129
Maxwell, A., 167
McAnany, H., 147
McCoy, C.B., 147
McDermutt, Representative, 16
McNeil, J., 100
Medicaid program, 7,9-11,10t, 12,12t
    described, 9
    recipients of, numbers of, 9,10t
Metsch, L.R., 147
MFIP. *See* Minnesota Family
    Investment Program (MFIP)
Mica, J., 32
Michael, R., 118
Michigan
    welfare in, 72-95. *See also* Welfare
        reform, in Michigan
    welfare reform in, 72-95. *See also*
        Welfare reform, in Michigan
Miewald, C., 5,163

Miller, M., 147
Minnesota Family Investment Program (MFIP), 34-35
Murray, C., 32
Music, bluegrass, 136

National Association of Manufacturers, 27
National Center for Health Statistics, 11
National Family Violence Survey, 144
National Forum, 6
National Health Interview Survey, 11
National Survey of American Families, 15
Nearby Labor Force (NLF), 40
New England town meetings, 130
NLF. *See* Nearby Labor Force (NLF)
Nonaged adults in United States, economic well-being of, gender differences in, 97-122
　effect of children on, 100
　increasing earnings of women effects on, 98-99
　marital status effects on, 99-100
　public income transfers effects on, 100-101
　study of
　　analysis of, 103
　　conceptual framework for economic well-being in, 102
　　data presentation from, 103
　　data source in, 101-102
　　descriptive statistics from, 103-107,105t-108t
　　discussion of, 117-120
　　findings of, 103-116,105t-110t, 112t-115t
　　historical background of, 98-101
　　methodology in, 101-103
　　OLS multiple regression analysis in, 107-116,109t-110t, 112t-115t
　　variables in, 102-103

Nonprofit sector, view of "the other America" after welfare reform, 69-95. *See also* Welfare reform, in Michigan

O Brother, Where Art Thou?, 135-136
Omnibus Budget Reconciliation Act of 1981,12
Osterman, P., 39
Otto Bremer Foundation, 190
Ozawa, M.N., 4,97,99,100

Packard Bell, 39
Palmquiest, R., 107,108
Peace Corps, 124
Peck, J., 169
Pereyra, M., 147
Personal Responsibility and Work Opportunity Reconciliation Act (PRWORA), 3,4,14,32,52, 57,63,65,70,71,72,74,89,90, 91,92,141,142-143,143,144, 145-146,147,166
Pesek-Herriges, P., 183
Pigeon, M-A, 42
Piven, F., 166-167,172
Poor
　assistance for, 15-18
　of Central Appalachia, described, 125-126
　in Clinton boom, 23-49. *See also* Clinton boom, staying poor in
　lack of commitment to, 11-15
Poverty
　among the elderly, 2
　Appalachian, 124
　Class and Inequality Division of the Society for the Study of Social Problems, 6
　in Clinton boom, 23-49. *See also* Clinton boom, staying poor in

culture of, in Central Appalachia, 132-134
driving out of, in private automobiles, 183-196. *See also* West Central Wisconsin Community Action Agency (West CAP)
    problem associated with, 185-190
health care for people of, in U.S., 7-21
and inequality, in U.S., introduction to, 1-6
inequality and, 28-30
myths related to, 165-168
power and, 28-30
public policy related to, 165-168
skills and, 28-30
War on. *See* War on Poverty
why it won't go away, 36-42
Poverty rates
    before and after government programs, 43,44f
    in U.S. (1960-2000), 25,25f
Power, poverty and, 28-30
PRWORA. *See* Personal Responsibility and Work Opportunity Reconciliation Act (PRWORA)
Pryor, F., 29
Public income transfers, effect on economic well-being of nonaged adults in U.S., 100-101
Public policy, poverty and, 165-168
Public supportive services
    and California welfare policy, 147-148
    CDA. *See* Critical discourse analysis (CDA)
    delivery system for, suggestions for improvements in, 158-160
    how participants are informed of, 141-161
    study of
        fear and distrust of caseworkers and system in general in, 155-157
        findings of, 149-158
        good caseworkers in, 154-155
        help from advocates other than CalWORKS caseworkers in, 152-154
        insufficient and insensitive information from CalWORKS caseworkers in, 150-152
        methodology in, 148-149
        sample in, 149
        suggestions to improve information given by caseworkers in, 157-158
    in welfare policy, context for, 142-144
Putting People First, 36

Quinn, T., 183

Raphael, J., 145,146
Raytheon, 39
"Ready for Work" program, 178
Reagan, R., Pres., 31,32,37
"Rediscovering the Other America: A National Forum on Poverty and Inequality," 5-6
Reagan-Bush era, 2
Reich, R., Sec. of Labor, 28
Reisch, M., 4,69
Richards, G., 27
Rifkin, J., 17
Rose, N.E., 143
Rural Action, 135
Rural and Appalachian Youth and Family Consortium, 127

Index

Salizzoni, F.L., 37
Salomon, A., 144,145
Sanderud-Nordquist, I., 183
Sarnoff, S., 123
Schaffer, D., 29
SCHIP. *See* State Children's Health Insurance Program (SCHIP)
School of Social Work, Loyola University, 6
Secretary of Health and Human Services, 33-34
Segal, E.A., 1,2,4,51
Segura, A.G., 5,141
Shaw, C., Jr., 167
Skid Row, 37
Skills, poverty and, 28-30
SNCC. *See* Student Nonviolent Coordinating Committee (SNCC)
Social Security Act, 8
  Title XIX of, Medicaid program, 7,9-11,10t, 12t
Social Security Administration, 3,56
Social Security benefits, 56
Society for the Study of Social Problems (SSSP), 6
Sociologists for Women in Society, 6
Sommerfeld, D., 69
Sommerfield, 4
Southern Appalachia, vs. Central Appalachia, 130
SSI. *See* Supplemental Security Income (SSI)
SSSP. *See* Society for the Study of Social Problems (SSSP)
SSSP Conflict, Social Action, and Change Division, 6
SSSP Family Division, 6
SSSP Health, Health Policy and Health Services Division, 6
SSSP Labor Studies Division, 6
SSSP Law and Society Division, 6
SSSP Sociology and Social Welfare Division, 6

State Children's Health Insurance Program (SCHIP), 56
Stock, C.M., 125
"Strategy of First Resort," 39
Stricker, F., 23
Student Nonviolent Coordinating Committee (SNCC), 127
Substance abuse treatment services/mental health services, 146-147
Supplemental Security Income (SSI), 9
Supportive services, how participants are informed of, 141-161
Survivors Insurance, 100

TANF. *See* Temporary Assistance to Needy Families (TANF)
Taxpayer Relief Act of 1997, 30
Taylor Institute, 145
Temporary Assistance to Needy Families (TANF), 14,91,100,101,143,146,188,190,195
"The Kentucky Way," 132,133
The Other America, 2,8,24,123,124
The Truly Disadvantaged, 53
Thompson, T., 33-34
Thurow, L., 42
Tilly, C., 166

UMW. *See* United Mine Workers (UMW)
United Mine Workers (UMW), 128
United Nations General Assembly, 98
United States, poverty rates in (1960-2000), 25,25f
U.S. Bureau of the Census, 119

Value added tax (VAT), 17
VAT. *See* Value added tax (VAT)
Violence, domestic, 144-146

Wall Street, 36-37
Wallin, S., 11
Wang, Y.T., 100
War on Poverty, 24,98,124,127
   health care coverage before, 8
WASPs, of Central Appalachia, 125
Weiner, J., 11
Welfare
   lived experience of, 172-174
   in Michigan, 72-95
Welfare policy, supportive services in, context for, 142-144
Welfare reform
   in Michigan, 72-95
      study of
         changes in agency programs in, 79,80t-81t
         changes in client demand and composition, 76-82,77t, 80t-81t
         client referrals in, 78
         data analysis from, 74
         discussion of, 89-90
         duration of client contact in, 78-79
         findings of, 76-89,77t, 80t-81t ,84t, 85t, 87t-88t
         implications of, 90-92
         inter-organizational activities in, 83,85t, 86
         limitations of, 74
         need for provision of emergency services in, 82
         relationships with governmental agencies in, 86-89, 87t-88t
         research methodology in, 72-75,73t, 75t
         sample characteristics in, 72-75,73t, 75t
         welfare policy and agency budgets in, 82-83,84t

political promises for, 51-67
   emergent themes from, 58t-61t, 58-65
   findings related to, 58t-61t, 58-63
   goal of legislative effort in, 60-62
   implications of, 63-65
   literature related to, 52-56
   methodology in, 56-58
   view of legislation in, 62-63
   view of problem and why reform is needed, 59-60
"the other America" after, view from nonprofit sector, 69-95. *See also* Welfare reform, in Michigan
   introduction to, 70-71
   literature review related to, 71-72
Welfare repeal, 32-36
Welfare-to-work households, 183-184
   criteria for, 187-190
   hypothesis of, 187-190
   problem associated with, 185-190
Welfare-to-work households transportation program, 187
Wellstone, P., Sen., 16,173
West CAP, 5. *See* West Central Wisconsin Community Action Agency (West CAP)
West Central Wisconsin Community Action Agency (West CAP), 5,183-184
   described, 184
   introduction to, 184-185
   overview of, 184-185
WESTconsin Credit Union, 192-193
WFRP. *See* Worcester Family Research Project (WFRP)
Wilder Research Foundation, 186-187
Wilson, W.J., 53
Wisconsin Works (W-2) households, 184

Withorn, A., 65
Wolman, W., 42
Wood, R.G., 99
Worcester Family Research Project (WFRP), 144

World War II, 53
Wray, L.R., 42

Yoon, H-S, 4, 97

SPECIAL 25%-OFF DISCOUNT!

Order a copy of this book with this form or online at:
http://www.haworthpress.com/store/product.asp?sku=4895
Use Sale Code BOF25 in the online bookshop to receive 25% off!

Rediscovering the Other America
The Continuing Crisis of Poverty and Inequality in the United States

___ in softbound at $18.71 (regularly $24.95) (ISBN: 0-7890-2097-1)
___ in hardbound at $37.46 (regularly $49.95) (ISBN: 0-7890-2096-3)

COST OF BOOKS _____	❏ **BILL ME LATER:** ($5 service charge will be added)
Outside USA/ Canada/ Mexico: Add 20% _____	(Bill-me option is good on US/Canada/ Mexico orders only; not good to jobbers, wholesalers, or subscription agencies.)
POSTAGE & HANDLING _____	
(US: $4.00 for first book & $1.50 for each additional book)	❏ **Signature** _____
Outside US: $5.00 for first book & $2.00 for each additional book)	❏ **Payment Enclosed: $** _____
SUBTOTAL _____	❏ **PLEASE CHARGE TO MY CREDIT CARD:**
in Canada: add 7% GST _____	❏ Visa ❏ MasterCard ❏ AmEx ❏ Discover ❏ Diner's Club ❏ Eurocard ❏ JCB
STATE TAX _____	**Account #** _____
(NY, OH, & MIN residents please add appropriate local sales tax	**Exp Date** _____
FINAL TOTAL _____	**Signature** _____
(if paying in Canadian funds, convert using the current exchange rate, UNESCO coupons welcome)	(Prices in US dollars and subject to change without notice.)

PLEASE PRINT ALL INFORMATION OR ATTACH YOUR BUSINESS CARD

Name		
Address		
City	State/Province	Zip/Postal Code
Country		
Tel	Fax	
E-Mail		

May we use your e-mail address for confirmations and other types of information? ❏Yes ❏No
We appreciate receiving your e-mail address and fax number. Haworth would like to e-mail or fax special discount offers to you, as a preferred customer. **We will never share, rent, or exhange your e-mail address or fax number.** We regard such actions as an invasion of your privacy.

Order From Your Local Bookstore or Directly From
The Haworth Press, Inc.
10 Alice Street, Binghamton, New York 13904-1580 • USA
Call Our toll-free number (1-800-429-6784) / Outside US/Canada: (607) 722-5857
Fax: 1-800-895-0582 / Outside US/Canada: (607) 771-0012
E-Mail your order to us: Orders@haworthpress.com

Please Photocopy this form for your personal use.
www.HaworthPress.com

BOF03